"The Object Lessons series achieves something very close to magic: the books take ordinary—even banal—objects and animate them with a rich history of invention, political struggle, science, and popular mythology. Filled with fascinating details and conveyed in sharp, accessible prose, the books make the everyday world come to life. Be warned: once you've read a few of these, you'll start walking around your house, picking up random objects, and musing aloud: 'I wonder what the story is behind this thing?'"

Steven Johnson, author of *Where Good Ideas Come From* and *How We Got to Now*

"Object Lessons describes themselves as 'short, beautiful books,' and to that, I'll say, amen. ... If you read enough Object Lessons books, you'll fill your head with plenty of trivia to amaze and annoy your friends and loved ones—caution recommended on pontificating on the objects surrounding you. More importantly, though... they inspire us to take a second look at parts of the everyday that we've taken for granted. These are not so much lessons about the objects themselves, but opportunities for self-reflection and storytelling. They remind us that we are surrounded by a wondrous world, as long as we care to look."

John Warner, *The Chicago Tribune*

"Besides being beautiful little hand-sized objects themselves, showcasing exceptional writing, the wonder of these books is that they exist at all … Uniformly excellent, engaging, thought-provoking, and informative."

Jennifer Bort Yacovissi, *Washington Independent Review of Books*

"… edifying and entertaining … perfect for slipping in a pocket and pulling out when life is on hold."

Sarah Murdoch, *Toronto Star*

"For my money, Object Lessons is the most consistently interesting nonfiction book series in America."

Megan Volpert, *PopMatters*

"Though short, at roughly 25,000 words apiece, these books are anything but slight."

Marina Benjamin, *New Statesman*

"[W]itty, thought-provoking, and poetic … These little books are a page-flipper's dream."

John Timpane, *The Philadelphia Inquirer*

"The joy of the series, of reading *Remote Control*, *Golf Ball*, *Driver's License*, *Drone*, *Silence*, *Glass*, *Refrigerator*, *Hotel*, and *Waste* (more titles are listed as forthcoming) in quick succession, lies in encountering the various turns through which each of their authors has been put by his or her object. As for Benjamin, so for the authors of the series, the object predominates, sits squarely center stage, directs the action. The object decides the genre, the chronology, and the limits of the study. Accordingly, the author has to take her cue from the *thing* she chose or that chose her. The result is a wonderfully uneven series of books, each one a *thing* unto itself."

Julian Yates, *Los Angeles Review of Books*

"The Object Lessons series has a beautifully simple premise. Each book or essay centers on a specific object. This can be mundane or unexpected, humorous or politically timely. Whatever the subject, these descriptions reveal the rich worlds hidden under the surface of things."

Christine Ro, *Book Riot*

"... a sensibility somewhere between Roland Barthes and Wes Anderson."

Simon Reynolds, author of *Retromania: Pop Culture's Addiction to Its Own Past*

"My favourite series of short pop culture books."

Zoomer magazine

"Bloomsbury's Object Lessons series never misses."

The Millions

BOOKS IN THE SERIES

Air Conditioning by Hsuan L. Hsu
Alarm by Alice Bennett
Ballot by Anjali Enjeti
Barcode by Jordan Frith
Bicycle by Jonathan Maskit
Bird by Erik Anderson
Blackface by Ayanna Thompson
Blanket by Kara Thompson
Blue Jeans by Carolyn Purnell
Bookshelf by Lydia Pyne
Bread by Scott Cutler Shershow
Bulletproof Vest by Kenneth R. Rosen
Burger by Carol J. Adams
Cell Tower by Steven E. Jones
Cigarette Lighter by Jack Pendarvis
Coffee by Dinah Lenney
Compact Disc by Robert Barry
Doctor by Andrew Bomback
Doll Maria Teresa Hart
Driver's License by Meredith Castile
Drone by Adam Rothstein
Dust by Michael Marder
Earth by Jeffrey Jerome Cohen and Linda T. Elkins-Tanton
Egg by Nicole Walker
Email by Randy Malamud
Environment by Rolf Halden
Exit by Laura Waddell
Eye Chart by William Germano
Fat by Hanne Blank
Glass by John Garrison
Golf Ball by Harry Brown
Fake by Kati Stevens
Football by Mark Yakich
Gin by Shonna Milliken Humphrey
Glitter by Nicole Seymour
Grave Allison C. Meier
Hair by Scott Lowe
Hashtag by Elizabeth Losh
High Heel by Summer Brennan
Hood by Alison Kinney
Hotel by Joanna Walsh
Hyphen by Pardis Mahdavi
Island by Julian Hanna
Jet Lag by Christopher J. Lee
Lawn by Giovanni Aloi
Lipstick by Eileen G'Sell
Luggage by Susan Harlan
Magazine by Jeff Jarvis
Magnet by Eva Barbarossa
Mask by Sharrona Pearl
Metronome by Matthew Birkhold
Mushroom by Sara Rich
Newspaper by Maggie Messitt
Ocean by Steve Mentz
Office by Sheila Liming
Oil by Michael Tondre
OK by Michelle McSweeney
Password by Martin Paul Eve
Pencil by Carol Beggy
Perfume by Megan Volpert
Personal Stereo by Rebecca Tuhus-Dubrow
Phone Booth by Ariana Kelly
Pill by Robert Bennett
Political Sign by Tobias Carroll
Potato by Rebecca Earle
Pregnancy Test by Karen Weingarten
Pub by Philip Howell
Questionnaire by Evan Kindley
Recipe by Lynn Z. Bloom
Refrigerator by Jonathan Rees
Remote Control by Caetlin Benson-Allott
Restaurant by Brian Duff
Rust by Jean-Michel Rabaté
Saxophone by Mollie Hawkins
Sewer by Jessica Leigh Hester
Scream by Michael J. Seidlinger
Shipping Container by Craig Martin
Shopping Mall by Matthew Newton
Signature by Hunter Dukes
Silence by John Biguenet
Skateboard by Jonathan Russell Clark
Sock by Kim Adrian
Souvenir by Rolf Potts
Snack by Eurie Dahn
Snake by Erica Wright
Spacecraft by Timothy Morton
Space Rover by Stewart Lawrence Sinclair
Sticker by Henry Hoke
Stock Photo by Simona Supekar
Stroller by Amanda Parrish Morgan
Swimming Pool by Hsuan L. Hsu
Taco by Ignacio M. Sánchez Prado
Traffic by Paul Josephson
Tree by Matthew Battles
Trench Coat by Jane Tynan
Tumor by Anna Leahy
TV by Susan Bordo
Veil by Rafia Zakaria
Videotape by Oana Godeanu-Kenworthy
Waste by Brian Thill
Whale Song by Margret Grebowicz
Wine by Meg Bernhard
X-ray by Nicole Lobdell

OBJECTLESSONS

A book series about the hidden lives of ordinary things.

Series Editors:

Ian Bogost and Christopher Schaberg

In association with

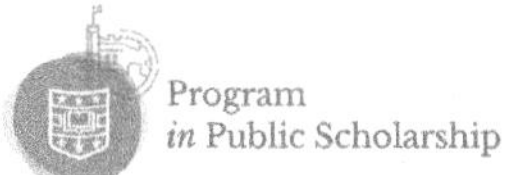

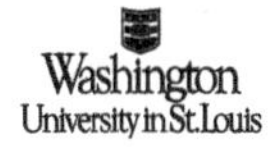

Lipstick

EILEEN G'SELL

BLOOMSBURY ACADEMIC
NEW YORK • LONDON • OXFORD • NEW DELHI • SYDNEY

BLOOMSBURY ACADEMIC
Bloomsbury Publishing Inc, 1359 Broadway, New York, NY 10018, USA
Bloomsbury Publishing Plc, 50 Bedford Square, London, WC1B 3DP, UK
Bloomsbury Publishing Ireland, 29 Earlsfort Terrace, Dublin 2, D02 AY28, Ireland

First published in the United States of America 2026

Series design by Alice Marwick
Cover illustration © Martina Pellecchia

A catalogue record for this book is available from the British Library.

A catalog record for this book is available from the Library of Congress.

ISBN: PB: 9798765135587
ePDF: 9798765135600
eBook: 9798765135617

Series: Object Lessons

Typeset by Deanta Global Publishing Services, Chennai, India
Printed and bound in the United States of America

For product safety related questions contact productsafety@bloomsbury.com.

To find out more about our authors and books visit www.bloomsbury.com and sign up for our newsletters.

For my mother, Maureen, who encouraged her four colorful daughters

CONTENTS

ILLUSTRATIONS

INTRODUCTION

At age eight, long before my adventures in inattentive babysitting, I joined the ranks of wayfaring laborers. My responsibility was great: hand-deliver dozens of Avon catalogs to neighbors' doorknobs. If they were pre-festooned with junk mail, I stuffed my wares into the mailbox, a practice I later learned was illegal. Every other week, I marched along our sidewalk-less streets to the addresses printed on sticker labels. Bagged catalogs hung from my arms like heavy plastic wings.

The Avon Lady lived across the street from the small home I shared with my three younger sisters (and, incidentally, mom and dad). A forty-something grandmother, she might as well have been anointed the Lady of Avon by some distant Empress of Pulchritude, crowned with an Aqua-Netted coif and robed in a rotating set of puffy-painted sweatshirts. Her powers dazzled by dint of her access to products. While the exterior of her white-shuttered ranch house nearly matched my own, its interior gleamed with peach taper candles, collectible thimbles, and, in the bathroom, a giant bottle of Skin So Soft that splashed all over when one stole a sniff.

Her name was Pat Rowland. When her husband Ronnie moved his motorcycles out onto the curb, it meant their garage would host a sale for discontinued Avon items. While my mom would rifle through perfumed roll-on deodorants, one of her few indulgences, I'd scrutinize a shoe box of lipstick samples, each about half the length of my pinky.

When Pat mentioned one summer that the neighborhood delivery was hard on her knees, I pounced. *I could be her assistant.* It seemed too good to be true: three or four dollars per route, and my pick of any leftover sample lipsticks. I already had door-to-door experience hawking my own homemade fragrances, lemon-scented "potions" I conjured with a chemistry set. Compared to shilling the fruits of my basement alchemy, this enterprise seemed no more arduous and likely much more lucrative. Over several seasons of St. Louis snowstorms and heat waves, I delivered the catalogs and stashed the cash in my jewelry box. The lipsticks were displayed over the trundle bed I reluctantly shared with my sister Beth.

As much as I admired my line of tiny totems snaking along the windowsill—which were repurposed as munitions for plastic Army troops to drop on toys below—I became transfixed at how I could transform *myself* with a careful swipe of a lipstick tube. This was an era in which lurid fuchsias were fading into a more sober array of browns, plums, and violets. A pale girl with dark hair that flew all over the place, I was hardly a paragon of late-'80s beauty, or what passed for that at my public grade school. I was bullied for an array of physical and sartorial deficiencies beyond my control: hairy legs, uneven bangs, off-brand denim, a scar above my lip earned in dodgeball.

Lipstick had a talismanic effect: it livened—or soured—my complexion immediately. A dramatic mouth on a pale face served to balance out my dark (uni)brow. Dusty mauve made my eyes look suddenly green; frosted lilac, on the other hand, made my teeth look downright daffodil. But the perfect lip color made me look—and feel—impossibly glamorous, as indomitable sauntering through the cafeteria as I felt during a math or spelling quiz. Given that, grade school through junior high, I was often the shortest kid in class, easily mistaken for years younger, this boost was no small feat. That my massive extended family censured any style that seemed too showy was just another reason that I, ever the girly gadfly, rebelled à la Revlon at an early age.

Though averse to beauty rituals herself, my mother consented to my new passion—amused, at times, by a brave new shade I chose to wear. In fact, when my sixth-grade social studies teacher, Mrs. Tayborn, shoved a brown paper towel in my hand and demanded that I remove my lipstick ("Plush Red" from Walgreens, if I recall) in front of the class, my mother was indignant. Despite her suspicion of any outsized zest for fashion and pop culture, she took the attitude that, so long as I performed well in school and never asked for spending money, I could do whatever I liked with what I earned myself.

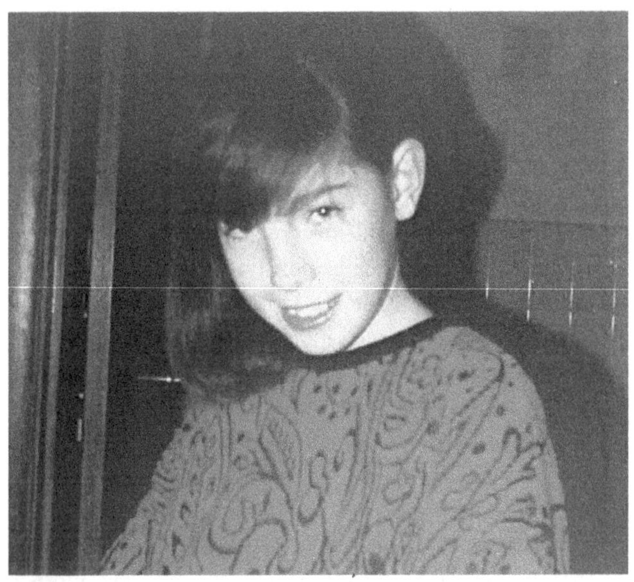

FIGURE 0.1 Author wearing red lipstick, c.1989.

And so it was that, years before the hormones of delayed puberty colonized my gymnast body, lipstick transformed my meek façade. It felt—and still feels—more natural to me than my naked mouth. It visually intensifies my too-loud laugh, too-deep frown, and too-quick smirk. It alerts the world to the most important part of my expressive face long before it moves to action. Without lipstick on, would I have gained the confidence to strut my stuff through the halls of five different schools from 1990 to 1994? Would I have (for better and, also, for worse) mouthed off so often—much to the chagrin of high school nuns, the frat boys vying to inebriate me in college, and untold authorities across adulthood?

Though I'd no idea of it at the time, I grew up during one of the flashiest—yet most conservative—periods of US history, when what Susan Faludi dubbed the "backlash" against Second Wave feminism was at its peak. "Publications from the *New York Times* to *Vanity Fair* to the *Nation* have issued a steady stream of indictments against the Women's Movement," her preface to *Backlash* emphasized in 1991. "They hold the campaign for women's equality responsible for nearly every woe besetting women, from mental depression to meager savings accounts, from teenage suicides to eating disorders to bad complexions."[1]

As I dimly remember it, the gains of the Women's Movement just a decade prior were often reduced to Tonight Show punchlines or (inaccurate) references to smelly hippies torching their brassieres. While Barbie ads preached that "girls can be anything," many in my generation developed the sneaky suspicion that this might not be the case.

And as the 1990s duly enlightened me, my penchant for lipstick was hardly universal. "I feel like a clown," my friend Steph would say when lining her mouth for the high school musical. "I never know what shade looks good on me," griped others (who, unlike me as a child, had apparently not repeatedly checked out the *Color Me Beautiful* series from the library). Those who shared my countercultural slant took to abrasive lip shades like black and bright blue—as evidenced in our sullen driver's license pics. By my senior year, I was both alterna-girl and lip color connoisseur, nicknamed "Eileen G'Smell-Good" by a guy friend for the trail of Bonne Bell Vanilla Frosting "Lip Smacker" sillage that wafted in my wake.

At the same time I savored the sobriquet, I was also experiencing what could only be called a secular feminist awakening. Why were friends at the rival boys' school applying for competitive, out-of-state colleges when I was chided for considering the University of Chicago? Why did girls primp for hours before homecoming when our dates rolled off the couch and put on a tie? Why did Sister Maureen scoff, "You've always been *ambitious*," when informed that I'd won a literary prize for a short story (a Salinger emulation, and, alas, the only award with which the National Endowment for the Arts has ever endowed me)?

Clearly, my love of lipstick—its aura of glamour, escape, and chameleonic personae—butted up against the reality that young women, me included, were so often treated like fonts of humility or mindless pretty objects. Did taking myself seriously as a thinker and doer mean renouncing one of the few things that had consistently (and affordably) given me everyday pleasure? Was I, like millions of other women, unwittingly participating in my own subjugation by painting my pucker a piquant pink?

The short answer: of course not. But as with most matters of gender, power, and femininity, the better, truer answer takes longer to come by and is as messy as a magenta smile at a summer rave.

Such is the ethos of this book. As lipstick itself[2] has materially transformed as an object, so too has its significance. The classic tube lives on, but as a relic of an older time in which conventional femininity was more requisite, and ergo more likely stifling. What lipstick means today has less to do with patents or packaging and more with how women, and others who identify as feminine, are permitted to style and package themselves—if they feel permitted at all.

More than thirty years from my Avon aspirations, I do not intend to endorse or decry lipstick, much less suggest that it means one thing to all women (or to anyone else). Rather, as a cisgender female, white Xennial of modest economic roots, I seek to reconcile my cognitive dissonance within the changing terrain of the twenty-first century, a time in which ideas about lipstick—and adornment in general—have noticeably shifted.

For Millennial and Gen Z women, lipstick hardly seems an everyday necessity (unlike, say, water bottles as heavy on the wrist as on the wallet). And yet lipstick—and lip stains, paints, glosses, and other forms of color—continue to fly off the shelves. In 2024, lipstick and lip gloss together netted some $785 million in the United States.[3] Lip "makeup" was the fastest-growing segment across both prestige and mass outlets,[4] fueled in part by a rise in Gen Z purchasing power.[5] This, despite the fact that, based on recent studies, nearly 30 percent of Gen Z US women identify as queer,[6] and 44 percent of the generation do not believe that gender is a binary.[7] Clearly, lipstick wearing today can't be tied exclusively to an army of hetero women chained to traditional feminine ideals or compelled to attract and gratify an omnipotent "male gaze."

So what, in the name of Maybelline, is going on?

In this book, I've no interest in rehashing the invention of the swivel-up tube or what shade means what in any given era. Others have already done so, some of whom did so very well.[8] Histories of lipstick are in fulsome supply, as are accounts of the "lipstick effect" as an economic metric. Neither account for lipstick sticking around even when many other feminine trappings have steadily declined (pantyhose, compulsory shaving, dyeing gray hair) as feminist priorities (equal pay and reproductive rights) have gained mainstream support—albeit lacking legal protection in many places.

Given that lipstick was one of the most iconic, if at times objectionable, objects of the twentieth century, it's no surprise that a lot of what was written about it then feels pretty retrograde—replete with bromides like "lipstick makes you feel like a woman" or, as the authors of *Read My Lips: A Cultural History of Lipstick* put it, the revelation that (surprise!) "all gay women were not the stereotypical, short-haired, leather-clad dykes that mainstream society had come to expect."[9] *Cringe.*

While some history is necessary for understanding the (many) reasons for lipstick's stigmatization and celebration, this book foregrounds the last two decades of the twentieth century and the first two decades of the twenty-first, during which women made unprecedented economic gains and the distance between assigned gender and sexual identity continued to widen. In all chapters, I explore how the act of painting one's lips continues to bear connections to class, race, gender, and other matters of identity and power. Aesthetically and politically, femininity doesn't mean what it did when I was a kid.

If, in the past, certain feminists conflated makeup with self-sexualization and internalized misogyny, many of today's self-described feminists—buoyed by the multi-billion dollar "wellness" industry—conflate vanity in general with "self-care." Once a sign of superficiality, looking good has been conveniently (and profitably) rebranded as a *moral* good.[10]

As skeptical of binaries as I am of "finger breathing" my way into better beauty sleep,[11] I'm inclined to see vanity as neither vice nor virtue. Like most pursuits in the name of beauty, it is relatively value-neutral. But just because something isn't inherently good or bad doesn't mean it can't lead to both good *and* bad outcomes for different people.

For someone like me—aiming to escape the conservatism of my childhood and the doldrums of desexualized femininity—lipstick has felt liberatory, prankish, and fun. But for someone made to feel less-than for lack of a painted mouth, lipstick could feel like an instrument of the oppressor, yet another way to make girls and women feel bad about themselves. For still others, especially those not summarily tagged "female" at birth, lipstick could be a way to experiment with femininity in ways otherwise stigmatized, even physically dangerous. No one's experience with lipstick can be invalidated by another's. When something is literally applied to the entrance of the mouth, a gate to gustatory and erotic pleasure, it's bound to have distinctly personal consequences.

For these reasons, the chapters that follow include not only my lived experience and critical analysis of lipstick as a cultural phenomenon, but the perspectives of women, cis, and trans—across age, race, class, and professional background—who graciously responded to a short questionnaire I created and distributed in late 2024.[12] While most examples will be Western and US-based, on occasion the book branches out to non-Western contexts. Between each chapter, handwritten vignettes about a salient lipstick memory or experience convey the wild panoply of ways in which this object has enlivened, burdened, delighted, and bemused across generation and identity.[13]

For many women surviving (and thriving) in the twenty-first century, "leaving the house without lipstick on" is no longer taboo. For that matter, neither is leaving the house *with* lipstick on for some who don't identify as women. Tossing expired ideas about femininity like so many tubes of melting wax, this book explores the ways in which self-adornment can be a source of play, pleasure, and transformation—and knock gender norms off balance.

1 PAINTED LADIES AND TAINTED MEN

Behold: a hand-carved vial containing a scarlet paste. Two inches by three-quarters of an inch, the stone vessel stands a smidge shorter than a tube of Clinique (in a similar shade of chlorite green), but taller than the plastic Avon testers that once fit my girlish hand.

In 2024, a team of researchers declared this Bronze Age artifact the oldest known extant lipstick—or, more precisely, container of lip paint. It is over 4,000 years old. According to the team's head archaeologist, the paste itself was identified as "exactly what one would expect in a modern lipstick": a mix of dye, oils, and vegetal waxes.[1]

Was it a woman who dipped her brush into its depths? A man? Someone who didn't identify as either? We can't really know. What we can deduce is that the object was designed to be handheld, fancy enough to flaunt in front of others, but light enough to be portable. The region in which this lip paint was found belongs to modern-day Iran, a country that has, since the 1979 Revolution, banned cosmetics for government workers, medical students, and women on state-run television. Despite these bans, Iran boasts the second largest market for cosmetics in the Middle East, and the seventh largest in the world.[2] Iran's compulsory hijabs have also intensified a desire to accentuate the one part of the body exposed to the public. For Iranian women, "faces continue to take on outsize importance," argues culture writer Zahra Hankir, "with makeup acting as a vehicle to elevate desires and ambitions."[3] To wit, a recent study of female-identified Iranian college students found that over half applied makeup three times a day,[4] compared to only ten percent of American women between 19 and 29.[5]

The most popular product for both groups? Lipstick.

"There is no known culture in which people do not paint, pierce, tattoo, reshape or simply adorn their bodies," asserted anthropologist Enid Schildkrout, curator of the 1999 exhibition *Body Art: Marks of Identity* at the American Museum of Natural History.[6] Just as we have inked our flesh, dyed our hair, and waxed our pubes since antiquity, people have tinted their lips for an array of aesthetic, spiritual, and practical reasons. Around 3500 BC, the Sumerians were the first to blend gemstones, wax, and oils to visually spice up their eyes and mouths.[7] About four centuries later, the Egyptians followed suit. As in Sumeria, painted lips signified economic status more than gender.[8]

It wasn't until the Greeks took over that painting one's face was conflated with femininity—and thus with the supposedly corruptive nature of artifice. Female sex workers wore red concoctions that boasted ingredients such as—wait for it—sheep sweat and crocodile excrement. For the first time in known Western history, women who *weren't* selling sex were discouraged from wearing lip color, as it was presumed to deceive men and imperil one's social status.[9] (Less concern was given for the kissability of reptile doo-doo on one's pucker.) The Roman empire restored a view of lip paint that had less to do with gender than class. High-ranking men took it up, such that tinted mouths lost feminine connotation.[10]

It would not be a stretch to say that, through much of history, when men elected to paint their mouths, legal regulations disappeared. Then, as arguably now, outlawing and stigmatizing lipstick had much to do with fears of feminine wiles and their sexual implications. In the Western modern period, whether the act of painting one's face was seen as self-sanctifying or self-degrading has continued to be a matter of economic status and power. Especially for women.

Western Lipstick Regulations and Taboos

When, in the sixteenth century, Queen Elizabeth I deigned to don a crimson mouth and alabaster cheek, it was a royal flex. When, over the next 300 years, English women of lower standing lacquered their lips, it was feared a form of witchcraft and almost criminalized.[11] When, in the early days of the United States, well-heeled "belles" imported "paints, patches, [and] powders"[12] to doll up for the DC social season, their faces were feted in fledgling national magazines. But when ordinary ladies wanted to partake in the frivolity of "rouging" their mouths and cheekbones, they were duly scolded—instructed on the virtues of a woman's "soul," [13] among other dull, intangible assets.

In the early decades of the United States, facial paint largely proved the province of the elite; the lower classes had to content themselves with the pretense that "goodness" was—implausibly—as good as good looks. "The press seemed to suggest that [lipstick] was fine for the socialite who had the time and resources to become adept at cosmetic use and social graces," explains Ilise S. Carter in her book *Red Menace: How Lipstick Changed the Face of American History*, "but still a problem to the everyday American gal, who should continue to rely on grit and piety."[14]

To put a fine (matte or glossy) point on it, for at least the first half of our nation's existence, for the few who already enjoyed economic power and cultural capital, self-adornment was tolerated, even lauded. But if a woman did not, wearing conspicuous lip color could be interpreted to mean that she was cheap, peddling herself as an object to be purchased and consumed. The message to women was essentially: be naturally beautiful (and notably virtuous!) to nab a decent mate, but don't be too sexy, lest your looks molest the menfolk.

We also shan't forget that, in the 1800s, painting one's face for flashy fun further conflicted with new female obligations to be paragons of morality. In the latter half of the century, the Victorian era championed women of all classes as a *civilizing* force: it was a woman's duty to enlighten and domesticate men who suffered (boo-hoo) from baser instincts. In the United States, the mission to tame the male beast was perhaps best exemplified in the Temperance Movement to abolish alcohol, a campaign almost entirely comprised of Protestant white women in sober attire.

Across the pond, Queen Victoria decreed lipstick "impolite," while the Church of England extolled the marriage bed as a repro-only zone. As such, female sex workers were deemed necessary to keep the wifely "angels of the house" properly resigned to tending to their bawling cherubs. While husbands could visit brothels to fulfill their needs,[15] horny wives had to toss off their haloes and fend for themselves (potentially dubbed hysterics if their rubbing rubbed authorities the wrong way). Contrary to common assumption, sex work in England thrived during this period *across* economic tiers, but it was only the underclass of sex workers whose cosmetics came to be seen as a means of disguising disease or "characteristic features which criminals exhibit openly."[16]

Similarly, depictions of the American West pitted "painted ladies" of the saloon against fresh-faced frontier wives[17] who dutifully maintained their complexions despite dust storms, drought, and diphtheria. We see this dichotomy

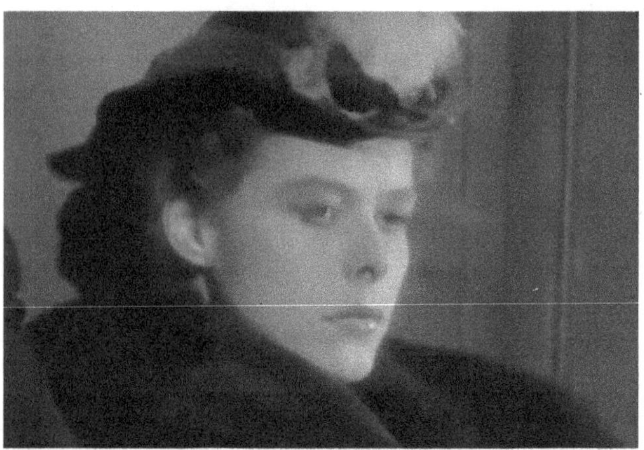

FIGURE 1.1 Louise Pratt in *Stagecoach*, 1939.

in twentieth-century representations of the period like John Ford's 1939 *Stagecoach*, in which scrappy sex worker Dallas (Clare Trevor) boasts a boldly painted lip while Mrs. Mallory (Louise Platt), her reluctant travel companion, appears much more subdued. A half-century later, the "Greeley Girls" depicted in Clint Eastwood's *Unforgiven* present a less glossy vision of sex work: no lipstick and fancy updos for these weathered women. However sympathetically Clint portrays them as characters, the Girls pale in comparison to the hero's saintly wife Claudia, who passes away before the film's story begins, but only after civilizing her drunken, murderous husband (after all, she'd fulfilled her life's sole purpose).

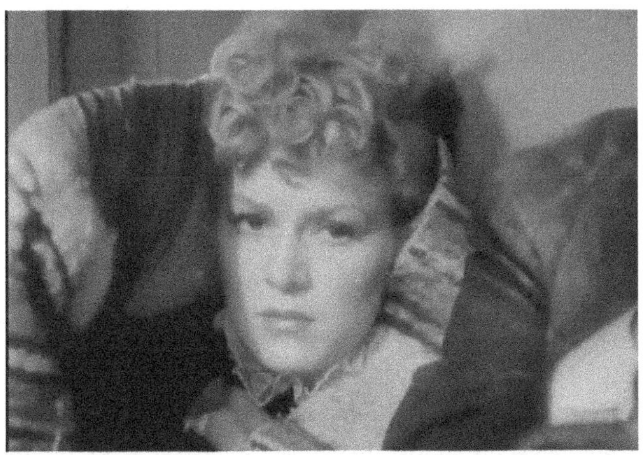

FIGURE 1.2 Clare Trevor in *Stagecoach*, 1939.

It was—and often still is—assumed that men are a witless species who cannot reliably divine whether the feminine beauty that attracts them is natural or contrived. Ergo, they must be protected from such weakness by women themselves. Painted lips on the wrong kind of woman—which is to say, a woman who lacks inherited wealth and aspires to upward mobility via run-of-the-mill hypergamy—can suggest visual deception, the exploitation of a man's naivete (if not his pocketbook). Female sex work itself wasn't federally banned in the United States till 1910,[18] but the connection between lipstick and the world's oldest profession has lingered far longer.

"No lasting love can be built on a lie, however trivial," warned Pittsburgh reverend Christian F. Reisner in the

Pittsburgh Press in 1912.[19] Much less was said about the ways in which women had been, for millennia, exploited by men, or to what extent men themselves found a painted pout particularly transfixing.

Sex Work Ambiguity and Declining Lipstick Stigma

In the twentieth century, lipstick's growing acceptance can be traced to the radically growing presence of women in public space toward the close of the century prior. The explosion of print media meant that women gained greater access to, and interest in, fashion and style norms; magazines and catalogs encouraged women to package themselves in the likeness of sundry trends to, presumably, attract male attention *and*, crucially, gain class status. With the dramatic expansion of mass print culture came new desires for an array of beauty products—lipstick just one of them.

How did lipstick shed (some of) its sex work stigma? Advertising. Print advertisers of the Victorian era purposefully smudged the line between the image of the sex worker and "respectable" woman to encourage potential female consumers to see themselves as connoisseurs of pleasure. "While moral narratives worked for a culture seeking to distinguish threatening sexuality from proper ladies," writes Jaclyn Reid, "the sexualized bodies of women in commercial culture were portrayed as pleasurable indulgences free of moral consequence."[20] Around the turn of the century, "imagery of the prostitute, as a symbol of pleasure, found a central function in the world of commodity culture."

But it wasn't crystal clear whether the lusty woman depicted was indeed selling sex—and the ambiguity of such figures in advertising wasn't just meant to titillate men. It was also a way to spark *new desires* among millions of women—at once encouraging them to indulge in certain products (and pleasures) once thought improper and, crucially, to see *themselves* as objects of visual consumption for others. In fashion mags and beauty ads, "such reveries of wealth and beauty, combined with sexual fantasies and desires, created a space for the prostitute as a subject of female desire and mimicry."[21] Sex sells—and, as advertisers quickly discovered, not just to randy Victorian lads.

Around the same time, due to innovations in lithography, color became a powerful means to attract the consumer gaze. Fashion and beauty marketing became that much more beguiling—with full-color illustrations and, later, color photographs. Conceivably, these color illustrations of fashionable women inadvertently *normalized* red lips as desirable, precisely because the woman depicted wasn't necessarily wearing lipstick, and precisely because lipstick itself wasn't often the object for sale. In an 1888 ad for "The Boltonian Under-Vest," a British girdle-like undergarment, the two young women feature unnaturally red lips. They also—naughty lasses!—are touching each other in a way that is more than a touch erotic.[22]

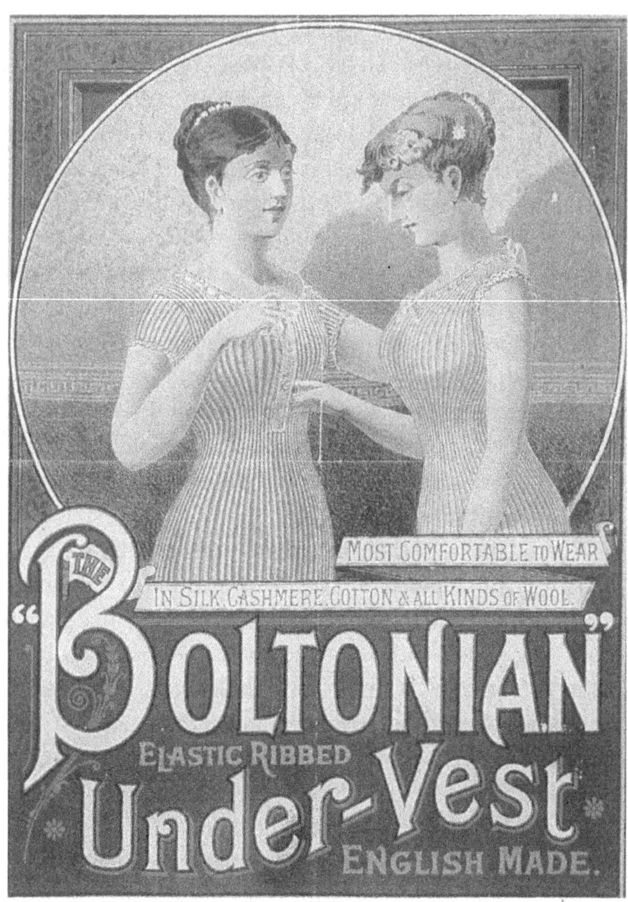

FIGURE 1.3 Color illustration for English Boltonian "Under-Vest," 1888.

Movie Mouths and Make-up as a "Creative Art"

Yet another big reason that lipstick[23] dropped some of its baggage: the explosion of motion pictures. As women, immigrants, and the working poor filled theater seats, American studios churned out fanzines that exhorted readers across social classes to identify with their favorite screen stars.[24] While good girls like Lillian Gish whimpered around in softer hues, the bold-lipsticked "vamp" emerged as a Hollywood archetype in the form of Ohio-born Jewish American Theda Bara,[25] whose lead turn in *Cleopatra* (1917) screamed cringey exoticism before Elizabeth Taylor was even born. Before they began incorporating photographs, movie mags like *Motion Picture Magazine* (1911–77) and *Photoplay* (1912–74) featured detailed, full-color renderings of celebrities from famous illustrators.[26] Once again, the hand-tinted nature of these images meant that one couldn't necessarily *tell* if the star was wearing lipstick or just inherited an enviably vibrant smile.

In 1910, Max Factor Sr. (Maksimilian Faktorowicz) invented the first foundation specifically for film actors (delightfully dubbed "Supreme Greasepaint"!). By the 1920s, Factor was Hollywood's preeminent makeup artist, marketing his $50 "makeup kits" to women who mostly couldn't afford them. His fifty-cent lipstick—about $9 today—proved an affordable luxury by comparison. Even more crucial to boosting makeup's rep, he shilled specific *techniques* that could enable the average woman to remake her face for the better. "What Max Factor has done for the Stars, he can do for you," reads a print ad from 1928.

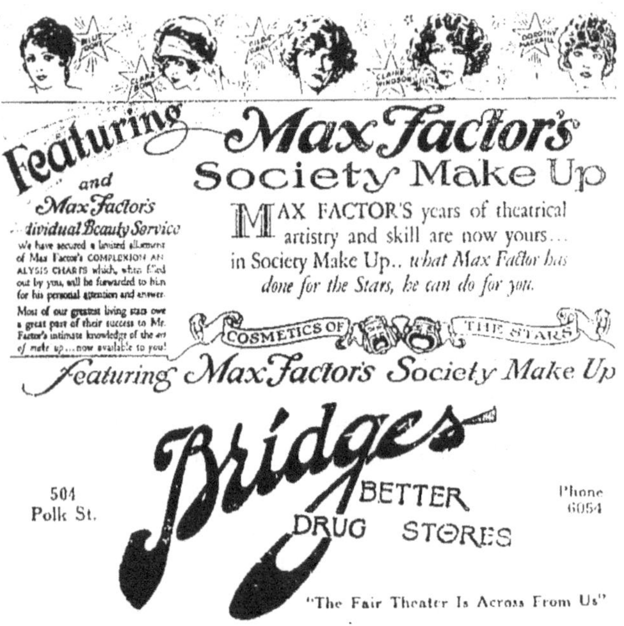

FIGURE 1.4 Max Factor ad, 1928, Courtesy of James Bennett.

The Polish Jewish immigrant perceived cosmetics as a "corrective art" that has transformative potential; it was about both concealing flaws and highlighting assets.

Penning the "Make-Up" entry for *Encyclopedia Britannica*'s 14th edition (1929–73), he wrote that "make-up serves to (1) cover blemishes; (2) provide the face with a smooth and even colour tone for the most effective photography; (3) clearly define the facial features for more visibly expressive action; (4) make the player appear more attractive; and (5) ensure a uniform appearance before the camera." In a more expressive vein, "[a]s a creative art, make-up enables the player to take on the appearance of almost any type of character. It can be his means of achieving a distinctive 'screen personality.'"[27]

Dubbing anyone who wore makeup an ungendered "player," Factor both reminded us of his brand's Hollywood cachet and encouraged a mostly female consumer base to identify as androgynous performers, capable of artfully cultivating their own feminine "personality" to others by identifying and then accentuating their most captivating features. His emphasis on the *camera's* presence also presumes that those wearing makeup in public might very well be captured by a lens—this nearly a century before iPhones would make that an inevitability.

But perhaps most vitally, the artificial properties of a made-up face were framed as a matter of creativity and self-determination. A woman could "take on the appearance of almost any type of character," and to do so wasn't deemed deceptive or licentious. Emulating onscreen sexpots, women could dabble in lipstick without fear of being perceived as an offscreen sex worker.[28]

Of course, that didn't mean everyone got away with it. In the Jazz Age, as in the Bronze Age, class and power mattered. American women nominally won the vote in 1919, but that didn't mean that all women *got* to vote; poll taxes, literacy tests, and other classist, racist measures prevented huge swaths of women (and men) from visiting the polls.[29] While the "right" to paint one's lips pales in comparison to suffrage, it's no surprise that poor and working-class women—and women of color—have long been subject to harsher judgment for their aesthetic choices. Not incidentally, these women have also been more likely assumed to be sex workers, with the additional hazards that entails. As I'll explore in a later chapter, lipstick stigma has lingered longer for Black and Latina women in particular. When a group is already hypersexualized by mainstream media, the repercussions for appearing flashy or colorful multiply in kind.

At the risk of painting the last 500 years of Western history with too broad a brush, the less economically secure a "painted lady" was presumed, the more she was feared to "taint" the men who beheld her. For women of lower status to remain "respectable," artifice had to be held at bay.

While the first half of the twentieth century witnessed the expansion of women's rights and the mass acceptance of painted faces, by the second half, the Women's Movement, along with a precipitous rise in high-earning female professionals, augured a reckoning with femininity and objectification. Lipstick—vilified a century prior as, at best "impolite," and, at worst, the mark of a "fallen woman"—was often labeled anti-feminist or self-sexualizing. Feminine adornment signaled capitulation to male desires, a lack of interest in joining the millions of other women who had become financially solvent through hard work and grit.

Of course, that's only one story.

"The Lipstick Revolution" and Mahsa (Jina) Amini

The idea that a "painted" woman is deceptive or dangerous certainly isn't limited to Western culture, and, indeed, has reached a fever pitch in modern-day Iran, the birthplace of the ancient lipstick vial 4,000 years ago.

Unlike the United States and other Western countries, for Iranian women, beauty rituals have never been considered vain or superficial,[30] and since the rise of the "morality police" who can arrest women for dress violations or "unchaste" behavior, lipstick has come to transmit political messages. Many Iranian women today see it as a weapon against an oppressive regime and as a way to honor their own bodily autonomy in public space.[31]

As Melody, an Iranian-American attorney and activist, explained to me, lipstick connotes "freedom, beauty, power, defiance against any people or governments that politicize religion or otherwise misuses power to control women." Recalling her visits to Tehran while growing up in the 1980s and 1990s, Melody noticed a sharp distinction between her own lipstick habits and those of her female family members. "My cousins tended to enjoy wearing plenty of makeup when we went out—and generally more than even I wore in the US—but I always refrained from wearing too much, including lipstick, to minimize any potential interactions with the morality police."

During the "Lipstick Revolution" of 2009, women flooded the streets across the country to protest the reelection of President Mahmoud Ahmadinejad.[32] Scanning the phrase in news headlines, I naively imagined thousands of brightly lipped women defiantly shedding their headscarves in public. But as extensive photojournalism from the protests attests, some women wore lipstick, but many did not. Most depicted donned a hijab. The "Lipstick Revolution" may have gestured to the most colorful aspect of the rallies, but had much more to do with women's lack of access to equal divorce, child custody, or inheritance rights.[33] The name that Western media ascribed to the protests could, indirectly, lead to a dismissal of their importance, just as anything aesthetic is often dismissed as feminine and therefore frivolous.

Lipstick isn't what the protests were primarily about, but lipstick *is* meaningful to Iranian women, and in ways that outsiders are likely to misunderstand. Melody shared how, in response to "how little makeup" she wore when visiting them in Tehran, some of her cousins "joked and teased" her by calling her "hezbolla-i" (as in, belonging to Hezbollah, a Shiite Muslim military group). "For them, wearing bold lipstick felt like a small sign of protest and defiance," she explained. "For me, it didn't seem worth it. I never wanted to get anyone else in trouble for something I did."

In 2022, the death of Mahsa (Jina) Amini under custody of the "morality police" launched a new wave of rallies that engulfed Iran and spread around the world. This time, women (and men) lifted signs with Amini's image, in which she is wearing lush red lipstick. Overnight, this shy 22-year-old salesgirl became an icon of resistance to restrictions on how a woman is permitted to appear in public.

Amini's personal Instagram account featured five selfies, in each of which she appears with a carefully made-up face and a bold red lip. While the official police statement

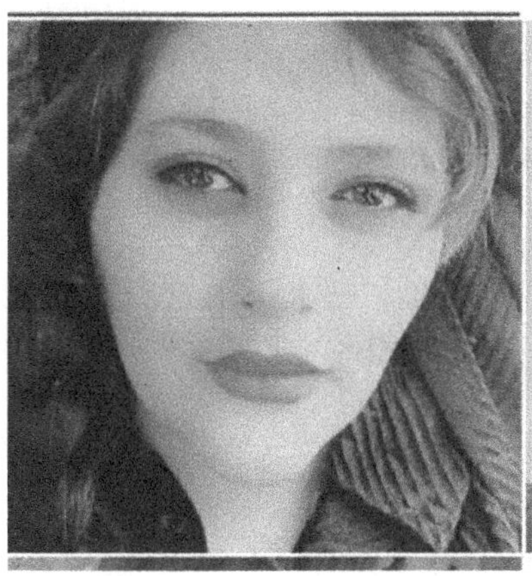

FIGURE 1.5 Mahsa (Jina) Amini's Instagram selfie, 2022.

reported that she was apprehended for not entirely covering her hair, I have to wonder whether she was wearing lipstick at the time of arrest. Fraught as the painted lip has been in the United States, it is profoundly so in Iran and other countries in which feminine adornment is regulated.

"I respect women who wear lipstick within dominant cultures that disapprove of lipstick," Melody asserted, "women in conservative religious societies, women in government and positions of power where makeup might be seen as frivolous or petty, trans women, and so on. They strike me as independent, defiant, affirming, confident, and powerful."

Independent? Defiant? Powerful? A far cry from the ways in which many feminists have seen lipstick in more secular societies like the United States and Europe, where feminine beauty is often seen as burden more than boon. Much of this difference in attitude has to do with how femininity is tied to either pleasing a man or teasing him—even when both are perceivably possible, even likely, at the exact same time.

In the West, the idea that lipstick is not only meant to stir male desire—and that, if it does, that needn't be degrading—is relatively novel. Whether concocted by marketers to peddle products or an honest reflection of a new zeitgeist, this shift has shaped the ways in which we understand femininity in the twenty-first century.

HANDWRITTEN STORY 1: MARGARET, BABY BOOMER

What words do I associate with lipstick?

Drama, chic, strong, vamp, starlet, 50s-60s, self-possessed, confident, eye-catching, bold, sexy, feminine, colorful, vibrant, fashion plate, girlie, bombshell, so many possibilities from barely-there nude gloss to in-your-face blood red, 50s housewife ads, tight-waisted dresses with heels, Greta Garbo, carefree, Somewhat obscene in drawing attention to your oral orafice, suggestive, cool being your own woman, lively, essential.

What words do I associate with lipstick?

Drama, chic, strong, vamp, starlet, 50s-60s, self-possessed, confident, eye-catching, bold, sexy, feminine, colorful, vibrant, fashion plate, girlie, bombshell, so many possibilities from barely-there nude gloss to in-your-face blood red, 50s housewife ads, tight-waisted dresses with heels, Garbo, carefree, somewhat obscene in drawing attention to your oral orifice, suggestive, coed, being your own woman, lively, essential.

2 PAINTED LADIES AND PAINTED MEN

For much of human existence, lipstick been feared for its potential to corrupt menfolk. Over my own lifetime, though, the tie between femininity, artifice, and attracting a man has become even more complicated—not least because Western women have achieved unprecedented (if still limited and uneven) access to financial solvency sans male support.

As determined by economist Martha J. Bailey, "The story is one of long-term, continuous progress, and slowing progress after 1990."[1] The decade that experienced the sharpest rise in American women's wages? The 1980s—not incidentally, the first decade I lived to stand and shimmy in. The jump in annual wages from 60 percent of men's to 71.6 percent happened in just ten years, reflecting "rapid increases in women's labor-force participation and their experience working for pay."[2] In this same decade, more than half of all bachelor's degrees were awarded to women, and about half of master's and 30 percent of doctorates. This meant that women—to be sure, disproportionately white and Asian women—acquired bigger earning potential at the exact same time that men, especially from the working class, were slipping in both wages and education.[3]

If fear of a painted face has stemmed in part from stigma over sex work, the fact is that women have gradually acquired a much wider array of ways to support themselves, many ways much more secure and profitable (not to mention legal) than the "oldest profession."

That said, apprehensions about unnatural or "artificial" femininity certainly haven't vanished overnight, even as the use of makeup by cisgender men spread from the counterculture to pop culture. Toward the end of the twentieth century, lipstick became popular among a range of male music celebrities—from David Bowie's Ziggy Stardust era in the early 1970s, to glam-metal band Poison and the English singer-songwriter Boy George in the 1980s, to acclaimed drag queen-popstar RuPaul in the 1990s. While each of these instances belied varying degrees of gender deviance (Bowie's and Poison's heterosexuality intact; Boy George's and RuPaul's homosexuality inferable), the ability of a painted face to visually flatter a man upset notions of lipstick as strictly for cis straight women. As Poison frontman Bret Michaels put it in 1987, "This makeup doesn't mean we're like women or we want to be like women. Do I look like a woman to you?"[4]

Amid such gender-bending on MTV, primetime American sitcoms like *Who's the Boss?*, *Growing Pains*, and *The Cosby Show* featured stylish matriarchs with ambitious

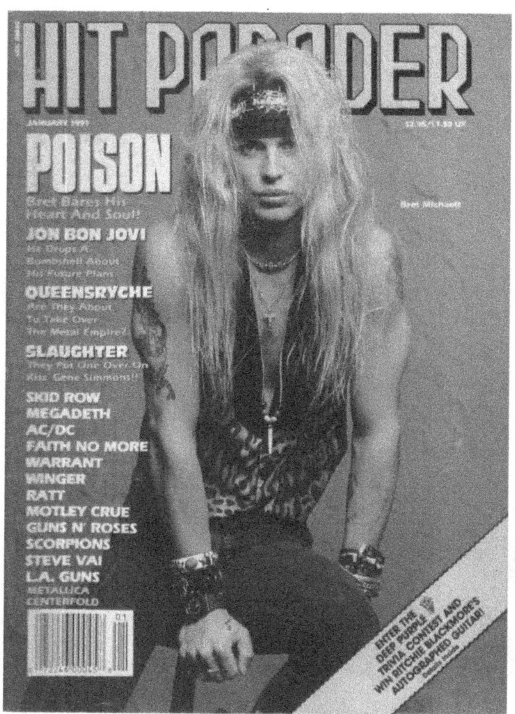

FIGURE 2.1 Poison's Bret Michaels, 1991.

careers (lawyer, journalist, different kind of lawyer). As a business exec in Mike Nichols's *Working Girl* (1988), Sigourney Weaver matched a "power red" sports jacket with a prominent lip. Contrast that with Melanie Griffith's girly receptionist, whose demure mauve smile literally pales in

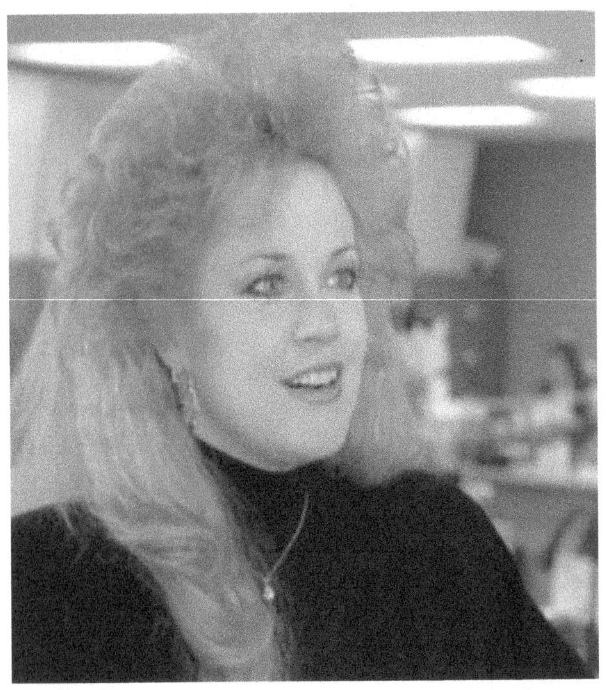

FIGURE 2.2 Melanie Griffith in *Working Girl*, 1988.

comparison. Gradually intensifying her look—and lip shade—as she gains power in the professional world, Griffith's heroine scrappily perseveres in this box-office hit, the title of which knowingly winks at changing conceptions of women's "work" from the oldest professions to the newest ones.[5]

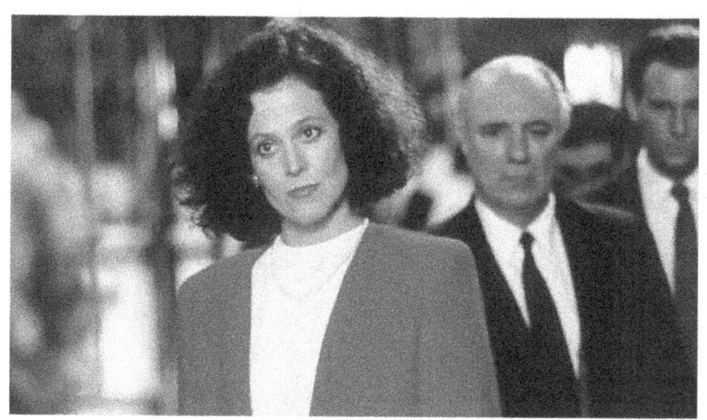

FIGURE 2.3 Sigourney Weaver in *Working Girl*, 1988

But in a world where women have learned the hard way that a strong will isn't always rewarded, a forward lip color can also backfire. Roseann, 71, shared with me that, as an Independent Arts Advisor and Strategist, she prefers a "good deep, red" for everyday wear, but worries it could look "too assertive in a more conservative, professional situation." She elaborated, "I've been told that I am sometimes 'scary,' so might tone it down to a deep rose or a mauvy nude. But lipstick, especially red, makes me feel dressed, ready, and stronger. Red's the color of passion, anger, blood, fire. And maybe I enjoy being 'scary'!"

Affiliations between lip color and professionalism have endured for Millennials and Gen Z today. "When I think of bold lipstick, I think of my bosses or women in business," Mya, a 30-year-old African American esthetician, told me. "It feels very grown up to me—which is crazy to say, my being a full adult!" Rather than connoting cheapness, a potent shade can do the opposite if one otherwise plays by the sartorial rules. In the 1980s and 1990s that meant comporting one's overall look to historically masculine standards—just one reason why pantsuits and shoulder pads overran the runway (Sigourney could face a running back!).

The 1980s also witnessed one of my (many) breaks with respectable girlishness. Around the same time, I was assigned a handful of Hail Marys after my first Confession (a reasonable penance for extravagant sins), I was in thrall to the *other* Madonna, the one whose red lips and bleached mane suggested danger, even sacrilege. With her dark roots and prescient boy brow, her version of femininity was unabashedly artificial. But her beauty, to me at least, felt incredibly real, her brash attitude genuine.

And so, a string of "True Blue" contradictions unspooled before me: What did "blonde ambition" mean, if your real hair was almost black? What did breakdancing in LA have to do with crossing the "borderline"? To be "like" a virgin meant that you *weren't* one—so why was Madonna bragging about it?

Who's That Girl? Madonna and Artificial Femininity

Mashing the vestiges of 1950s glamour with CBGBs punk rock, the Material Girl was enamored of, well, materiality.

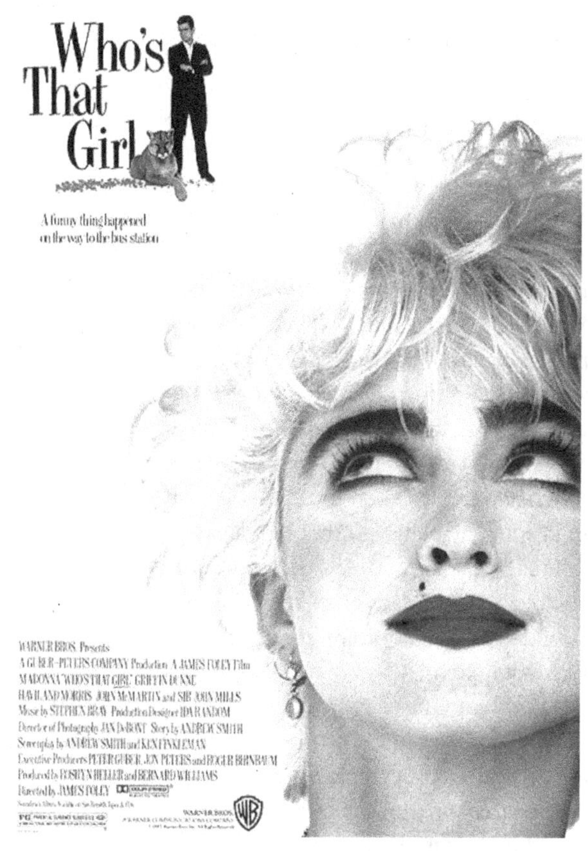

FIGURE 2.4 *Who's That Girl* movie poster, 1987.

She was glittering surface, black rubber bracelets, flagrant fuck-you fakery. She was hardly virtuous and often seemed to bask in just how prankish she was. "Who's That Girl" begged the title of her second movie (that, even with its PG rating, I wasn't permitted to see). Dominating the white poster, Madonna seemed to simultaneously look up at her male suitor and roll her eyes at him. Her brick red lips were lined so sharply they resembled a Rubik's Cube.

That same year, in the finished basement of neighborhood It Girl Shannon Crecelius, wearing layers of her mother's discarded lingerie, my sister Beth and I performed to Madonna's "Papa Don't Preach," rating each other for originality and skill. With each revolution of the vinyl record, we straddled armchairs, collapsed on the carpet, spun with our hands in our tangled bowl cuts. We were six and seven and having a blast—perhaps me even more so, as I suspected the lyrics were verboten to repeat. "I made up my mind … I'm keepin' my baby!" Beth, predictably, belted the next day at the supermarket. "Where did you hear that!?" our mother inquired. While Madonna's red lips may have symbolized rebellion against patriarchs, it was Mom who Whac-a-Moled our Madonnaphilia.

But no amount of parental surveillance could have kept the Queen of Pop out of our house. Jutting her elbows, hips, and conical Gaultier breasts into Reagan-era TV screens, Madonna championed makeup's role in creating a version of selfhood that flouted the rules of feminine decorum. Scavenging signifiers from the underground dance club

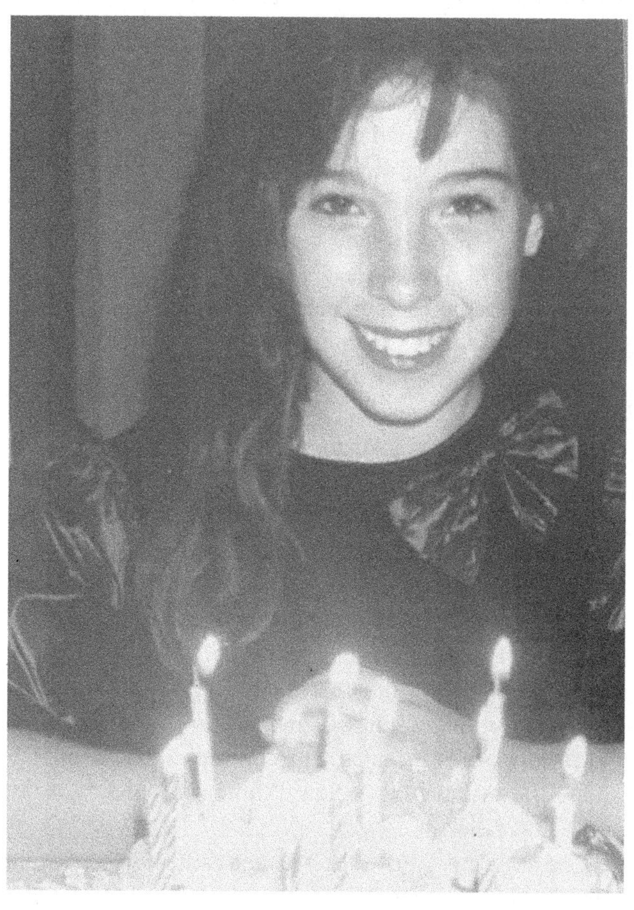

FIGURE 2.5 Author wearing lipstick for birthday party, c. 1992.

scene, drag queens, Marilyn Monroe, and other culture milieux, she was less celebrated for her voice or dance skills than her presence as a performer, a chameleonic capacity to transform herself into wildly different "types" of women.

In contemporary parlance, a lot of this borrowing would be called cultural appropriation—and rightly so. Madonna borrowed[6] from marginalized communities to boost her street cred and edgy demeanor, and often, in doing so, erased the subcultures creatively responsible. When I was pantomiming the choreography for her hit single "Vogue" in 1990, I had no clue that I was really parroting queer communities of color that invented the dance form at least a decade prior.[7]

At the same time, Madonna was the first female pop star I followed who openly celebrated the ingenuity of gay culture[8]—during a period in which open homophobia was on the rise. At the end of a decade in which the AIDS pandemic (and subsequent national neglect) had ravaged the gay community, Madonna was also among the first mainstream stars to directly address the crisis. Her 1989 album *Like a Prayer* (another hit I missed out on, though the video for the hit song was popular even if, like me, you didn't have cable) included an insert with facts about HIV and AIDS, encouraging "safer sex" among a largely ignorant youth population.

Like many my age in the late '80s and early '90s, I was taught that being "gay" meant you were practically guaranteed to get AIDS, spread it to others, and die.[9] Terrified that I could be one of these unfortunate gays—did I want to *be* Madonna? be *with* Madonna? both??—I was both alarmed by the pop star's deviance and duly intrigued with its possibilities. (Yes, I was one of those who snuck a peek at her 1992 *Sex* book at my local public library.)

Long before I learned about "lipstick lesbians" or sexuality as a spectrum, Madonna's hyper-stylized, irreverent take on femininity seemed vaguely connected to breaking taboos that lurked in every corner—not unlike the ubiquitous "dope" dealers D.A.R.E. warned us about. Why did the men in her videos seem to want each other more than her? What power did beauty give her if her chief aim wasn't nabbing a man?

In her videos and concert performances, Madonna courted an audience that admired her not on the basis of sexual desire, but from a position of allegiance to her shamelessly pro-sex, pro-kink identity. At the same time, she abetted a cosmetic culture that rejected the virtuous, naturally beautiful (usually white) woman as the feminine ideal. Was Madonna Ciccone conventionally attractive? You bet your rosary she was. But like her gym-chiseled physique, her face, hair, and overall appeal felt (wo)manufactured, artfully contrived.

For Madonna's 57-show "Blonde Ambition" tour in 1990, she wore MAC's "Russian Red" lipstick, and the fledgling Canadian brand took off as a result. Founded by hairdresser Frank Angelo and his partner, makeup artist Frank Toskan, Makeup Art Cosmetics (MAC) was the first major brand to celebrate makeup on nonwhite, often genderqueer faces, even when marketing *to* a largely white cisgender consumer base. They were also among the first to overtly claim—in their very name—that putting on makeup could be a form of *art*, not conformity to fashion or method of self-improvement.

MAC, Sephora, and the Right to Be "Pretty"

Like Max Factor, a brand still popular at the time, MAC presented lipstick and other cosmetics as a means to creatively transform oneself. Unlike Max Factor, the "artist" at MAC's helm wasn't a straight cisgender male makeup artist to the stars, but an openly gay male couple who tossed the idea that makeup was limited to straight women vying to look pretty for straight men. Early spokespersons for MAC's Viva Glam campaign—from which all profits have been donated to HIV/ AIDS organizations—included RuPaul, k.d. lang, Boy George, Mary J. Blige, and Missy Elliott. By the late 1990s, MAC had yanked lipstick out of the dainty grip of white, straight women and placed it on the faces of drag queens, lesbians, and people of color.

Was I, as a teenager, inspired to save my IHOP and Steak 'n Shake tips to purchase MAC lipstick? Hardly. For many aspiring fashionistas, the cost of a tube of Viva Glam was prohibitive: at least twice that of the drugstore brands. You

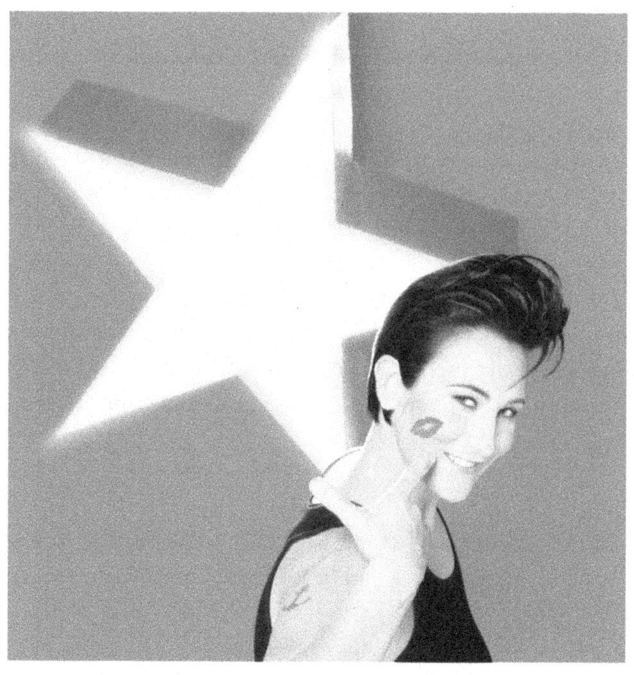

FIGURE 2.6 k.d. Lang by David LaChapelle for MAC Viva Glam, 1997 ©David LaChapelle

could smack your lips with a daring (or darling) MAC look if you were able—and willing—to pony up $12 in 1994, and $13 in 1996. Before eBay commerce and the Amazon Aughts, you also had to live in a city with either a MAC store or department-store kiosk.

By the turn of the twenty-first century, Sephora had tilted the needle even further in the direction of creative and personal experimentation. No longer did one have to rely on the beauty "experts" at department store counters—who were often made up like anchor women or pageant contestants—to try out products. At Sephora, you could sample anything yourself, and the salespeople who worked there—and who wore makeup—were typically *not* all cisgender straight women. The idea that one could transform oneself not to conform to gendered expectations, but to *thwart* them, felt just a tiny bit radical. At least in certain ways, Sephora was quietly ahead of its time in terms of genderqueer inclusivity.[10]

Outside of midnight *Rocky Horror* screenings, the first time I saw lipstick on anyone who wasn't a ciswoman was at a San Francisco Sephora in 2002, when I absconded from a Model UN conference with a redheaded hippy representing Botswana. Beguiled by the transwomen of color working there, I asked one about her glittery eye shadow. After poring over what seemed an infinite selection of shades and shimmer, I ultimately selected a mini-eyeliner and a $20 pot of red lip gloss.[11] While I was convincing myself that this jelly-like substance was worth a Thomas Jefferson, my hemp-necklaced friend filched a tester.

New Yorker columnist Jia Tolentino was Sephora-struck around the same time, when she was in grade school. Her Houston store was, unsurprisingly, more conventional than the one I visited in San Francisco's Union Square. "Sephora was right by the Victoria's Secret in the mall," she writes. "[T]he stores seemed aimed at the same audience (women, not eleven-year-olds) and at the same goal—making oneself alluring to men."[12] But Tolentino's aspirations were less to lure a pre-pubescent boytoy than to partake in the rituals connected to pretty privilege. "I had wanted to be pretty since the moment I grasped that being so meant more easily procuring affection from my peers and approval from my superiors," she recounts, "something that's as true in pre-K as in the workplace."

True as it is that girls are unfairly valued for beauty much more often, and much earlier, than their male counterparts, Sephora is a brand that, like MAC, has long reframed "prettiness" as available to those across the gender spectrum. On one (manicured) hand, such inclusivity clearly expands their customer base, leading to greater profit. On the other, the company's outwardly progressive ethos reflected diverging attitudes about femininity in the twenty-first century. If lipstick isn't worn exclusively by heterosexual ciswomen, to what extent is it meant to simply make oneself "alluring to men"? And do straight dudes even really *like* all that glitter?

Art vs. Artifice

Where an overtly painted mouth was once a signifier of sex work—and so, by extension, a visual ploy to lure the male gaze—queer icons like Madonna and RuPaul, along with makeup brands like MAC and Sephora, have nudged the meaning toward gender-bending and artistic agency. Art, unlike artifice, suggests expression rather than deception. And yet art, by definition, is inherently artificial—as in, made and produced by humans rather than occurring "naturally." The difference between art and artifice isn't one of form so much as moral consequence: art uplifts where artifice, ostensibly, corrupts.

Over the last two decades, makeup artists have launched a bevy of eponymous brands—among them Pat McGrath, Patrick Ta, and Charlotte Tilbury—joining longstanding names like Bobbi Brown, MAC, and Kevin Aucoin. It comes as no coincidence that, alongside this "artistic" branding, "lip paints" flooded the beauty market by the 2010s. Packaged as tubes of pigment meant to be applied with a separate brush (requiring its own maintenance), lip paints are less convenient than a tube of lipstick but make up for it in pigment intensity and conceptual appeal. To embrace the act of "painting" is to see one's face as a veritable canvas, one's hand as exact and dexterous: one is not a mere "makeup artist," but an *artiste*. By comparison, a cylinder of colored wax feels banal, a throwback to the days in which lipstick was obligatory, floating around one's bag or purse for frequent touchups.

But does the intent and process of lipstick application change its effect on others? That is, if I *feel* like an artist brushing on Fenty's Stunna Lip Paint, does that mean I actually am one?

Regarding the visual and literary realm, critic Becca Rothfeld argues that once art is valued for function over aesthetics, it is no longer art. "The moment that an artwork is directed at some handy end … the second it acquires the kind of 'point' that can be trotted out in precious homilies," she writes, "it ceases to be what it is and becomes a mere implement, no more exalted than a broom or pedometer."[13] Accordingly, "the aesthetic resides in excess and aimlessness, in wants that spill far beyond the narrow bounds of need."[14]

Applying Rothfeld's argument (perhaps generously!) to the realm of self-beautification, when a person—usually a woman—feels the *need* to paint herself, whether to attract male attention, or, as Tolentino put it, "procure affection from … peers and approval from … authorities," then at best it can be a creative take on a practical goal. It cannot be art. Lipstick is art when the goal and effect is not to achieve a "handy end" but to conjure a look that exceeds functionality. Perhaps that is why lipstick often feels the most artful when it is applied outside the context of heterosexual attraction or *Working-Girl* careerism.

Of course, that doesn't mean that cosmetic brands haven't taken off with "paint" nomenclature, squeezing out its ambiguity to boost sales across genders. And of course, that doesn't mean that lipstick cannot be "artistic" on cis, straight women. "It can be a powerful thing to use make up in ways that challenge the social standard of beauty," artist and arts educator Livia, 28, shared with me. "I think a bold lip-color like black or green can feel radical and freeing from the male gaze. When I wore bold colors when I was younger, it felt like I was wearing them just for my happiness."

Glossier and "Good" Beauty Choices

The notion that lipstick *isn't* for lassoing male sexual attention—or attracting sexual attention at all—has seduced new minions in the twenty-first century. No brand has fostered this idea more fully than Glossier, the brainchild of ne plus ultra Millennial girlboss Emily Weiss. The direct-to-consumer beauty brand exploded around 2014 and championed the cosmetic wearer as an *artist-creator,* not a passive consumer. Rather than tie its products strictly to a particular part of the face, Glossier deliberately touts its wares as malleable and multipurpose, maximizing the prospect of creative decision-making. What goes on your lips could also go on your cheeks—or your eyes (why not?).

Purposefully pronouncing her brand to rhyme with "dossier," Weiss further suggested that enhancing one's face could boost one's career prospects (even more important to those who joined the workforce post-Great Recession). "Skincare is essential," proclaimed early Glossier ads. "Makeup is a choice. (Make good choices.)" Perfecting—and exploiting—such rhetoric in its subway banners and Instagram posts, Glossier knew that a lot of young women in the 2010s did not feel that lipstick—or any cosmetic, for that matter—was mandatory for appearing hip or professional. But if you're already in a habit of making "good choices" with one's life (perhaps to pay off that college debt) why not do so with makeup as well?

Adolescents and teens at the time were also caught up in Glossier mania—in no small part due to how the brand embraced social media and e-commerce for marketing and sales. As Helen, 20, shared with me, "Glossier packaging was less gaudy than other makeup at the time. Visually and in design, Glossier competed with other brands not by adding more visual stimuli, but by seeming to take it away."

How best to shill lipstick to those who believe they don't need it? Call it something else. "Cloud Paint," one of their most popular products, debuted on Instagram before Glossier's website was even up. Easily mistaken for a tube of oil paint, the product is meant to be applied to the lips and face with one's fingers. As a moniker, "Cloud Paint" marries the semi-transparency of floating water vapor with something heavy, manmade, and staining. That, too, is by design. Prefer watching wispy clouds to contouring one's cheekbones? Cloud Paint is for you. Desire a "naturally" garnet grin rather than a garish grimace? Buy yourself some cumulus pigment!

Today's Cloud Paint product page features a young Black model with bleached brows and a cascade of wavy braids. Her flawless skin appears makeup-free—save for a rosy flush to her cheeks that matches an ever-so-subtle sheen on her lips, both offset by a sheer, fuchsia turtleneck over a white

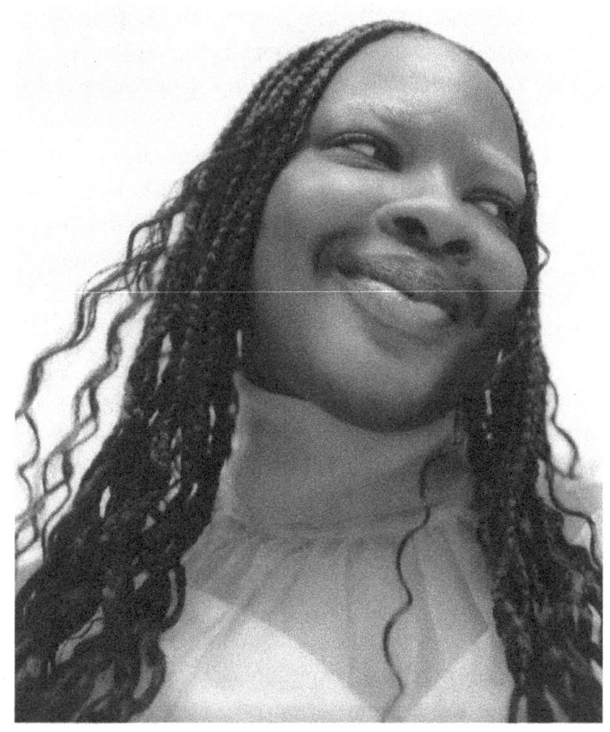

FIGURE 2.7 Glossier Website, Cloud Paint Product Page, 2025.

bra. "Ibti wears Cloud Paint in Soar," the caption reads. With her soft smile, lifted chin, and gaze directed out of the frame, she seems like a woman unburdened by beauty dictums and ready to float toward deserved bliss.

The accompanying description heralds Cloud Paint as "the most user-friendly blush + bronzer under the sun"; it is, providentially, "so natural it's like your skin made it." Being "user friendly" means that you don't need any brushes or sponges to put it on, and that "each shade is sheer enough to blend and layer without going overboard." Suggesting that the product for sale will in no way conceal or detract from the "natural" appearance of its wearer, Glossier has proven just how much consumers will shell out to a company that not only accepts but *affirms* their quirks and flaws—if only superficially. (And at $22 for .33 ounces, that's no small amount.)

On Planet Glossier, electing to color one's face brings cosmic pleasures all its own, even (or perhaps especially) when said makeup is barely visible. In their 2022 "You Look Good" campaign,[15] a three-minute video presents a montage of men, women, and nonbinary people—diverse in race, size, gender persuasion, and, to some degree, age—sharing when they last felt like they "looked good." Each model, many of whom do not seem to be wearing make-up of any kind, articulates a context for "looking good" that is both relatable and mildly idiosyncratic. "I like to cook," says a ravishing young woman of South Asian descent, upon which the phrase "You look good cooking" appears in all-caps font, affirming it as true. "Happiness and joy and passion make you look good," asserts a gender-nonconforming person in a septum ring and spectacles. "'You look good' is self acceptance," says a young Black man.

A middle-aged woman shares how important it is to tell her sixteen-year-old daughter that she looks good; "it makes her feel loved." At the end, the words "YOU LOOK GOOD" appear onscreen repeatedly as each model tells the viewer that we, also, evidently, "look good."

And who doesn't want to feel that way? The absurdity of the ad—the models can't see us, so can't know what we look like—is eclipsed by Glossier's virtuous message: looking good isn't about appearances, but just about how one *feels*. Of course, if this were true, no one would need to paint their face with tinted clouds.

"[T]he aesthetic preference for a natural beauty look that disguises its true level of effort … owe[s] a debt to Glossier," writes culture critic Diana Heald.[16] In Glossier's shadow, many other brands have since rolled out "lip paint" as part of a makeup palette. In 2017, *Allure* magazine declared lip paints "the ultimate liquid lipstick/lip gloss hybrid,"[17] ticking off products that resemble Dick Blick booty more than makeup. Bobbi Brown's top-selling "art stick" resembles a chubby crayon, bringing to mind hours coloring unicorns—or Hot Wheels—during childhood.

Rebranding lipstick as an *art* tool carries multiple connotations. "The way you had to blot [Cloud Paint] across your lips and face was like finger painting," Helen recalled of her tween years using the product. "Not only did it turn you into an artist, but it drew you back to nostalgic ideas of playing with your mother's makeup."

Haus Labs and Painted Kindness

Stealing a page from Cloud Paint, Lady Gaga's Haus Labs cosmetic line, which launched in 2019, sells "Hy-Power Eye, Cheek & Lip Pigment Paint" in shades from sapphire to peach. Brighter and more intense than its Glossier kin, each tube is even tinier at .23 fluid ounces. But once again consumers are encouraged to "mix paints to create custom shades" (again: *you* are the artist!), even though the product itself seems tougher to apply ("apply to face or body with a brush and allow product to set").

On the "About Us" section of the Haus Labs homepage, no fewer than seven unconventional models surround Gaga as though posing for a class photo.[18] One masculine-looking platinum blond boasts blue eyeliner and shimmery pink lips; a glamorous femme septuagenarian sports silver tresses and a matte red mouth; two plus-size models, one of dark complexion and one conspicuously freckled, don shiny, open-mouthed grins. Gaga herself looks somewhat demure, her mouth magenta against a neutral face. "We are a collective of the Haus of Gaga," proclaims the first paragraph, "a collective of creatives, scientists, and innovators, who give you beauty tools for clean artistry. Kindness and inclusivity, forever."

In this vision of inclusive beauty, lip color—like any other face paint—is available to anyone who can afford the price of admission ($24 for Pigment Paint or $22 for Le Lip Crayon). “We aren’t serving looks,” one thumbnail reads. “We’re serving self-love.” It’s an amped-up version of MAC’s Viva Glam campaign from the 1990s, lifting the queer parlance popularized by *RuPaul’s Drag Race*. Painting one’s lips isn’t just about creative expression; it’s about being a stable, compassionate person (one who is, conveniently, quite pleasing to look at.) Women can wear lipstick; men can, too; so can those who identify as neither. As hyperbolic (and appropriative) as “serving self-love” may very well be, this messaging can disinhibit male-identified audiences who want to experiment with makeup but are hesitant to do so. The pleasures of self-adornment should be something to which all genders ought to have access without fearing shame or judgment.

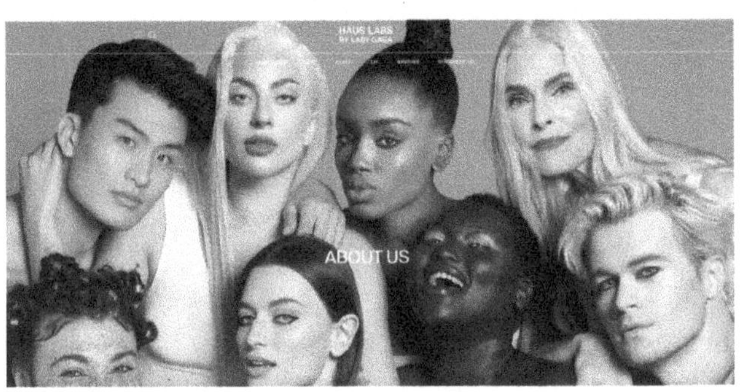

FIGURE 2.8 Haus Labs Website, “About Us” Page, 2025.

In her 2017 book *Man-Made Woman*, trans theorist Ciara Cremin unpacks the "sensual alienation" experienced by men discouraged from exploring or exhibiting femininity. Of course, frippery hasn't always suggested emasculation for Western men, nor has masculine authority required aesthetic restraint: just look at the Founding Fathers! But "in the [modern] westernized form of masculinity," she claims, "men are alienated … from the sensory stimulations, pleasures of craft, and expressions of individuality associated with the feminine gender."[19] Cremin celebrates feminine dress and makeup as a source of singular pleasure—one that most cis-men never get to experience. "Faces and bodies are the primary canvas on which our creative capacities find expression and … paint is an index of what as a society we have collectively accomplished," she writes. "Masculinity is a pallet full of greys. Colour is drained, textures are coarsened, the bouquet is scent-free. It is a miserable selection that men are nonetheless proud of."[20]

But as Cremin also notes, it need not be that way. As is clear from Haus Labs and other brands featuring male models brandishing lip color, lipstick has, in the course of a half-century, evolved from conventional feminine signifier for cisgender, heterosexual women to a means of honoring the "self," regardless of gender identity or sexual persuasion.

How did this shift square with feminism, with its ever-cresting and troughing waves? The answer depends on what "feminism"—as a political movement and personal ethos—sees as its fundamental foe.

SIDEBAR #1: THE PESKY ENDURANCE OF PUBLIC HIGH SCHOOL LIPSTICK BANS

In 1921, Pearl Pugsley was sent home from her Knobel, Arkansas, high school for wearing lipstick and powder. With her parents' support (and likely resources), this unfortunately named teen sued the public school district for violating her "civil rights."[1] On the heels of the Nineteenth Amendment, which gave (mostly white, middle class and affluent) women the right to vote, Pearl's right to self-beautify was reframed as itself a feminist act. "I'm going to fight … to uphold women's rights to use all reasonable means to look their best at all times," she professed to national media.[2] For a red-hot second, the pandemonium surrounding the case reached a fever pitch, prompting headlines across the country and, according to Pearl's mother, "a ton of letters" sent by sympathetic female readers. Unsurprisingly, the Arkansas Supreme Court dismissed the case. Even less surprisingly, women's rights organizations didn't exactly rally for the cause. In fact, with the Eighteenth Amendment passed, quasi-feminist Temperance groups shifted their efforts from banning booze to maligning makeup.[3] No wonder so many lipsticked flappers saw their flasks *and* faces as the mark of a rebel.

Almost a century later, we take for granted that young women can turn up to school with lips bedecked in Wet n Wild or Fenty Beauty. But what about young men? In 2018, Abner Garcia, a student in the Alvin Independent School District (ISD) outside Houston, Texas, was asked to remove his lipstick or face in-school suspension. In a dazzling act of defiance, Garcia refused; in turn, his friend Jasmine Richards launched a Change.org petition that read as follows:

> Alvin ISD has a dress code policy in place that includes several gender-biased policies such as preventing boys from wearing makeup and earrings (both things that girls are allowed to wear). These policies are based entirely on outdated and sexist gender standards. Prohibiting boys from wearing makeup because makeup is "only for girls" also prohibits them from expressing themselves in what is supposed to be a safe environment.

Prompted by the petition, the district dropped the ban within the year. Appearing on local television news to comment on the policy change, Garcia appears in a striped black T-shirt, pink lip gloss, mascara, and a buzz cut, explaining calmly that "everyone should be able to express themselves." Against the colorless space of the school parking lot, Garcia's brazen self-adornment is—to my eyes at least, the *definition* of rebel glamour. Alvin ISD should print his likeness on the school's annual calendar.

Jasmine Richards does not appear in the television spot, which is too bad, as she epitomizes a genuinely heroic disregard for gender norms—no matter the conservatism of the Lone Star State. Texas is not exactly friendly to teen gender-nonconformists; in 2023, it became the largest state in the country to ban gender-affirming care for transgender youth.[4]

For their part, the ACLU has made clear that "a public school may not enforce a dress and grooming policy that prohibits boys, and only boys, from wearing nail polish, or imposes rigid restrictions on hair length based on gender. Such dress codes marginalize non-binary, transgender, and gender-nonconforming students, and ultimately send the message that these students do not belong."[5]

For Dorothea, a transwoman who grew up in Connecticut in the early aughts, lip color was a rite of passage during a critical time in adolescence. "When I was in my early teens, my mom gave me a lip balm that was slightly pigmented, and

I found it thrilling the way it would modify my appearance ever so slightly," she explained to me. "That was the first time I wore makeup, and it allowed me to experiment with gender presentation and selfhood. I was at a private high school with strict 'boys' and 'girls' dress codes. In an environment where even hair dye wasn't allowed, lip balm, and later glosses, allowed me a bit of freedom to express myself."

Handwritten Excerpt #2: Maurice, Older Millennial

Recently I thought to myself, "I am going to master the colour Red for my lips."

Red is the iconic colour for lipstick, but because it is so bold, you have to get it just right. And my lips are noticeable & so, the pressure is on.

Recently, I finally nailed it with small strokes & patience. I stood in front of my bathroom mirror, & applied coverage to the intensity you want & that your face can handle. I did that for a good 25 minutes (tip: play music so you don't notice how long it is taking you to get ready).

When I was done it was perfection — the perfect lip for my face, so perfect I decided I wasn't going to kiss anyone or eat anything that night because I didn't want to fuck it up.

And I didn't.

Recently I thought to myself, “I am going to master the color red for my lips.”

Red is the iconic color for lipstick, but because it is so bold you have to get it just right. And my lips are noticeable, so the pressure is on.

Recently, I think I finally nailed it with small strokes and patience. I stood in front of my bathroom mirror and applied coverage to the intensity that I wanted and that you can handle. I did that for a good 5 minutes. Tip: play music so you don’t notice how long it is taking you to get ready.

When I was done it was perfection. The perfect red lip for my face, so perfect I decided I wasn’t going to kiss anyone or eat anything that night because I didn’t wanna fuck it up.

And I didn’t.

3 LIPSTICK FEMINISM AND STICKY PLEASURES

In 1999, when I arrived at the September meetup for Students Against Sexism in Society (cheekily dubbed "SASS"), likely wearing a dELiA*s tee and violet corduroys, I stood out like a frosted macaron at a table of Nutri-Grain. My whimsy felt like an affront to those who took feminism (and fiber) more seriously. No one in the room was wearing makeup. No one was wearing colorful or patterned clothes. If hair was dyed, it was dyed jet black, not an uneven burgundy like mine. Would lacquered lips out me as an informant for the other side—and if so, who was that, exactly?

I never returned to SASS.

My sophomore year, I dialed down the girliness with black emo glasses and Dickies trousers. From my short-lived stint as a pre-med student to my Tokyo study abroad,

I distanced myself from any trend that seemed too frilly, for fear of seeming vapid. In social circles, I also avoided the term "feminism"—not because I rejected its tenets, but because I feared being mistaken as a militant, man-hating, or gloomy killjoy (or perhaps all three!). While I labored on a senior thesis exploring the incongruity between French feminism and Japanese women's literature, as a college-radio host I mocked folk rockers Dar Williams and Ani DiFranco for their granola feminist sincerity. I was a walking contradiction—or hypocrite, depending on the lighting.

All the while, ditching lipstick would have felt like betraying my face: my dark brows floating lonely above my nose with nothing below to balance them out. While I kept my attire mildly edgy and my hair a notch darker than it grew in, I rotated between a crimson lipstick and a series of sparkling glosses. By graduation it was obvious that, as a parvenu to the literary scene, my penchant for the feminine could undermine my creative and academic ambitions. But looking the part of a lady academic—bare face, shapeless clothes, a splashy scarf if one wanted to get wild—simply was not *me*. Visual abundance and eclecticism had always brought such joy, and I wasn't willing to give it up, even if it might boost the impression that I was worthy of being called "Professor."

The idea that anti-feminine style itself could bear Puritanical, even misogynistic, roots never crossed my mind.

The Beauty ... Myth?

"A woman without paint is like food without salt," scoffed Naomi Wolf in her 1990 *The Beauty Myth: How Images of Beauty Are Used Against Women* (many years before she leapt onto the conspiratorial laps of the alt-right).[1] *The Beauty Myth*'s central thesis was that, while women gained more professional ground in the seventies and eighties, beauty standards were becoming ever more impossible to achieve. During the decade that I came of age, then entered college, Wolf's manifesto was flying off the shelves, propelled by snappy aphorisms like: "Women are allowed a mind or a body, but not both." An undoubtable (and redoubtable) hottie at 28, Wolf clearly had no problem seeing herself as both a body *and* a mind. Her point was that lipstick—like all forms of "paint"—was so obligatory for women as to be offensive when absent, a naked fry among seasoned pomme frites.

A hassle to maintain (if easy to apply), it's easy to see why lipstick has ruffled the feathers of feminists like Wolf (who wouldn't have been caught dead in a boa in the first place). Nothing like a bright lip color to declare one's face a decorated surface, the visual equivalent of "Look at me: an object!" from a scarlet megaphone. In fact, the very phrase "lipstick feminism"—touted by some to mean a celebration of femininity as strength—was first wielded by a feminist in 1994 to *dismiss* women who were thought to be "light on issues, heavy on vanity."[2]

It's also tough to dismiss Wolf's thesis when considering the conservatism of beauty media in the 1980s, when lipstick was often dubbed "a primal need" and "the one cosmetic women can't live without." In an era when many women still considered makeup necessary for leaving the house, lipstick was the most efficient and obvious way to appear made up. Foregoing lipstick was thus one of the simplest ways to flout patriarchal authority.

When I was growing up, the idea that a woman could wear bold lipstick *and* be an intellectual flummoxed both feminists *and* certain men. As music critic René, 58, recounted to me, when she worked at a popular used record store in 1989, her Boomer boss told a coworker, "See that girl across the aisle checking the understock? The one with all the lipstick? Would you believe *she's* in a PhD program?" Looking back, René was "mostly mad that he used the phrase 'all the lipstick,'" *not* that he said something so dismissive. ("I have always applied lipstick in precisely the optimal quantities," she reported.)

Even if a woman isn't *trying* to court male attention, she might still feel that's the message that lipstick sends. Nora, a 43-year-old filmmaker, shared that "playing down femininity" is a must in her male-dominated field. "In some contexts, it's delusional for women to wear lipstick and simultaneously demand not to be flirted with by the opposite sex," she reasoned. "To those who claim to be 'wearing lipstick for themselves,' perhaps you are, but you still have to acknowledge that it has an effect on others."

For that exact reason, Cynthia, a 35-year-old Chicana professor, generally avoids colored lipstick because it seems to affect how seriously she's taken by strangers. "I'm objectified more when I'm wearing it," she observed. At the same time, Cynthia doesn't find lipstick in tension with identifying as a feminist, especially given the toll of feminine "purity" tests. "In my conservative Christian upbringing, women that wore noticeable makeup were considered whorish or worldly," she explained. "To me, lipstick says, 'I do not conform to your ideals of modesty and so-called natural beauty.' Even though makeup is viewed as a traditional expression of femininity by the rest of society, I still get joy from protesting beauty ideals I grew up with."

When asked about her first memory of wearing lipstick, Cynthia recalled being cast as a "sinner" sex worker in a religious play held by her church youth group. "I was the only girl who had developed breasts, so of course I started associating having small breasts and no makeup with being good and Christian-like," she explained. "When I discovered feminism, I worked hard to unlearn these teachings and spent many years wearing lipstick and makeup as a way of healing."

While Cynthia's introduction to lipstick may seem extreme, her experience highlights how persistent, and harmful, the lipstick/sex-work connection can be among certain Christian communities. But not all women with religious backgrounds were raised to see makeup as so loaded. "When I was growing up, lipstick wasn't an issue at all to my feminist identity," Aisha, a Gen X columnist from Texas, told me. "The parts of myself that felt in conflict were identifying as a feminist and a practicing Muslim. Eventually, I reconciled these layers of my identity when I read Third Wave feminist writers and feminist Islamic scholars."

The Polarization of Small Pleasures

Lauren Gurrieri and Jenna Drenten, two of many feminist scholars to examine the politicization of women's personal consumption choices, claim that, like high heels and shapewear, lipstick is a "polarizing marketplace icon … simultaneously associated with both women's autonomy and oppression."[3] While I agree that all three consumer categories are polarizing, I'd counter that lipstick differs in significant ways. Lipstick has not been known to cause pain to its wearer or to gradually compromise the physiognomy of the body (ask any podiatrist about stilettos). Unlike everyday shapewear (Spanx the most popular, though corsets have recently enjoyed a ribboned resurgence), lip color also does not typically lead to irritated skin, problems breathing, or acid reflux. Lipstick also tends to be cheaper than shoes or Spanx, and more accessible to low-income women for whom small pleasures can be few. How likely is one to feel "oppressed" by a $4 tube of Walgreens lipstick when scrimping to pay for insulin at the store pharmacy?

But what is a pleasure for some has also, crucially, been a burden to others. Barb, 70, a retired nurse and current dance teacher in rural Missouri, views lipstick "as just too much trouble." Deborah, a retired librarian and self-identified feminist who came of age during "the early '70s counter-culture revolution," temporarily gave up lipstick when she "became a hippy" at fourteen. Margaret, a visual artist and professor, submitted "a passionate thesis" for her undergraduate honors degree in 1975, "on makeup as a masking, negative abomination." Fifty years later, she joked to me, "I was wearing lipstick when I wrote it, a natural-looking gloss. And the strange thing is, I adore lipstick now." For many Boomer women in their youth, lipstick seemed a sexist throwback in a time that demanded radical change.

This stigma against lipstick—as being fussy, self-sexualizing, and visually gratuitous—has lingered for many who, like me, came of age in the late twentieth century. Froggi, a queer, cisgender "child of the '80s," unabashedly justified her lipstick-loathing. "It looks gross, it tastes gross, it smells gross," she declared, "and even if none of the above were true, the feminine coding and associations of lipstick are all at odds with the identity I want to project."

Dorris, who is 40, Black, and genderfluid, also eschews lip color for its sexist connotations. "By wearing lipstick or lip gloss, I am 'playing the part' of some kind of gender expectation which really doesn't align with my everyday life," they explained to me, adding, "I see wearing lipstick or lip gloss as nothing more than a performance for others, not a form of personal expression."

When viewed as a signifier of (presumably) passive womanhood, lipstick is, quite logically, a tool of the oppressor. In a world where adornment is required to gratify male expectations—of a girlfriend, wife, secretary, or, on rarer occasions, colleague or even boss—it makes sense that reapplying Revlon would feel utterly retrograde.

But do we still entirely live in that world today? And who is that "we" to begin with? In most feminist literature, "we" has meant educated white women who likely have the means to support themselves sans a male patron (otherwise known as a husband). But "we" should also include Latinx, Black, South Asian, and other women whose cultures tend to prize vibrant expressions of femininity. "We" should also mean folks who reject the gender binary. And "we" should also mean working class women who, lacking financial and cultural capital, might need to rely on their appearances for economic survival.

The more power dynamics are surveyed across a diversity of experiences, the less lipstick (or any other affordable, anodyne beauty tool) feels categorically oppressive. I've no right to discredit Boomer and Gen X notions of lipstick as another vestige of self-sexualization, much less claim that lipstick, or any other cosmetic, is automatically "liberating" or "empowering" for all. In the periods in which many women came of age and battled sexism—of a type I have (fortunately) endured in more diluted doses—rejecting the rudiments of being "pretty" for public consumption had clear political goals. To many women, it still does. I respect these goals. I admire them. But I'm not convinced that, a quarter of the way into the twenty-first century, lipstick has to mean the same thing it did in the twentieth.

Uncle Sam's "Dim View of Beauty"

When did anti-lipstick attitudes first manifest in feminist circles?

In the United States, feminist aversion to makeup can be traced back to nineteenth-century suspicions of ornamentation and glamour (both affiliated with sex work, to be sure). In her 2005 book *Fresh Lipstick: Redressing Fashion and Feminism*, Linda M. Scott emphasizes that American censure of feminine adornment originated among elite, white, East Coast women who rose in rank in the 1800s: Elizabeth Cady Stanton and Susan B. Anthony among them. The "feminists led by Anthony and Stanton belonged to the most aggressive and powerful cultural subgroup in industrializing America," she writes, "the Yankee Protestant descendants of the pre-Revolutionary aristocracy."[4] These affluent, educated white women advocated both for dress reform (no more corsets!) and for the right to vote. They also tended to overlook, or even erase, the views of women with inferior class status or less ascetic aesthetics.

Provocatively asserting that "feminism's anti-beauty ideology serves the interests of the few at the expense of many,"[5] Scott goes to great lengths to show that feminist elites were *not* the only ones rallying for women's rights at the time: tens of thousands of middle-class, working-class, and immigrant women contributed to the cause. In addition, activists like "Fanny Wright, Victoria Woodhull, and Emma Goldman argued passionately for the rights of women to have beauty and pleasure, especially in sexual expression."[6] The anti-frippery attitudes of early feminism did not represent the whole movement; they are rather the aesthetic fruits of the "Stanton–Anthony" tradition.

Anti-lipstick feminism can also be traced back to Victorian notions of the "natural" woman, a font of replenishable goodness and domestic civility. Reprinted in the East Coast literary mag *The Albion*, an essay by English journalist E. Lynn Linton did not mince words about the colorful "Fashionable Woman" of the era: "She will not try simplicity of living, natural hours, wholesome occupation, unselfish endeavor, but rushes off for help to paints and cosmetics, to stimulants and drugs, and attempts to restore the faded freshness of her beauty by the very means which further corrode it."[7]

In ways not unlike the "wellness" craze of the early-2020s, beauty was conflated with a "wholesome" lifestyle, a sign of virtue rather than an evanescent creation of one's own making. Linking "paints" to "stimulants and drugs" would have further shored up classist *and* racist images of sex work and opium dens, both which turn-of-the-century media made out to imperil women—specifically white ones. With our country's history of white supremacist beauty standards, it should be no surprise that anxieties about lipstick and other makeup often have racialized backdrops. To *The Albion* writers, it is the "natural" purity of white women that is "corrode[d]." White virtue, beauty, and femininity are essentialized in one fell swoop.

As Ilise S. Carter deftly puts it, "White, Protestant, American popular culture has always fetishized the concept of 'self-made.' When it comes to selling the idea of transforming and improving one's self appearance, [early] women's magazines simultaneously endorsed the idea that this was possible *and* the idea that 'true' or 'natural' beauty was borne of temperance, piety, and even patriotism."[8] No wonder that so many American women—whether paging through *Vogue* in 1925 or scrolling through TikTok in 2025—endure the emotional whiplash of "you are beautiful if you are *good*" and "you could be *more* beautiful if you take these steps . . . ." Platitudes like "everyone's beautiful in their own way" further fail to convince when stacked against the ongoing reality of lookism.

For women who identify as feminists, the virtues of looking good can grow ever more fraught. "American feminism takes a dim view of beauty," Scott claimed in 2005.

"Across the spectrum of academic and popular literature, feminist writers have consistently argued that a woman's attempt to cultivate her appearance makes her a dupe of fashion, the plaything of men, and thus a collaborator in her own oppression."[9] In the past two decades, many feminists and gender activists *have* challenged anti-beauty and anti-feminine dicta—from academics like Merri Lisa Johnson, Hannah McCann, Amber Musser, and Jennifer Baumgardner to cultural influencers like Natalie Wynn and Alok Vaid-Menon.

But Scott's argument resonates with my own experience of ostracism—in college and beyond—from certain (but certainly not all) feminist groups and people. "In every generation," she writes, "the women with more education, more leisure, and more connections to institutions of power—from the church, to the press, to the university—have been the ones who tried to tell other women what they must wear in order to be liberated."[10] As someone from a lower-middle-class background, and the only one of my sprawling family to pursue academia, I've often felt a keen pressure to assimilate by adopting a more subdued style. If I were less constitutionally disagreeable, I probably would've done it. But I'd rather be a gadfly in a glittery dress (and matching lip) than conform to what feels bland and predictable.

Will "every generation" of privileged women, as Scott puts it, proceed to school those below in the same classist way? There are signs that highly educated young women today don't necessarily conflate liberation with anti-feminine aesthetics. As Sophie Lewis recently put it in an essay for *Harper's*, misogyny includes "the denigration of the femme subtype of femininity as void of intellect, strength, and even valid will."[11] Just as it is backward to conflate a woman's worth with her beauty, it is also backward to suggest that any pursuit of beauty is a flight from self-worth.

As Kaylei, 21, relayed to me, "I've never felt like looking 'feminine' has ever seemed in conflict with 'being feminist.' On the contrary, I feel that 'being feminist' means dressing the way one wants, including feminine, and being respected regardless." For those reticent about the rise of "choice feminism"—the idea that anything a woman chooses to do is automatically feminist because she chose it—Kaylei's response might feel too easy, a way to reap the benefits of feminine presentation while also applauding oneself for feminist virtue. It's a bit of having your cake (-flavored lip gloss) and eating it too (let's hope it's non-toxic!). But her attitude may have more to do with her generation's increased awareness that adopting an androgynous, even masculine, persona and aesthetic comes with baggage all its own—forcing some women into trappings that feel no more authentic than a jock strap. "When I was first learning about feminism in middle school, the pictures in the history books showed women 'dressing like men'—wearing pants and such—and not wearing make-up," Kaylei explained. "I couldn't tell you why, but at the time, I had already known that feminism was about female empowerment, not just about women wearing pants."

Of course, for many mid-twentieth-century icons (Katherine Hepburn and Frida Kahlo both come to mind) wearing pants was one way of appropriating masculine authority. Doing so granted a kind of power that, with so many acceptable clothing options for women today, can be easy to overlook. When *Legally Blonde*—a film many of my college students have seen multiple times—hit the screens in 2001, the repercussions of being "too blonde" (i.e., feminine) in an academic or professional setting were comedically exposed for their classist, even misogynistic overtones. When feminists join the "pretty police" force, they reinforce harmful beliefs that a feminine woman cannot also be smart.

The Sticky Pleasures of "Femvertising"

Feminists have also critiqued lipstick, and cosmetics in general, for upholding a narrow feminine ideal that benefits a patriarchal beauty industry. While it's debatable how much of the industry has been run by men, it is undeniable that beauty brands profit from female insecurities. Thin lips, acne scars, puny brows? There's a product for that! These days, there are hundreds. But it's also rash to conclude that women pursue these tools solely out of flagging self-esteem.

Despite its reputation for preying on hang-ups, beauty brands have been on the vanguard of "femvertising," which, rhetorically at least, does the opposite: wielding pro-woman messaging to market goods regardless of their connection to feminist goals. Relatively recent examples include Dove's 2004 "Real Beauty" campaign, and Procter and Gamble's 2014 "#LikeAGirl" videos, the latter of which generated more than 90 million YouTube, Facebook, and Twitter views in its first two months.[12] With their moving montages and feel-good voiceovers, these campaigns suggest that women and girls can be anything and do anything—so long as they purchase the proper product first.

In 2019, L'Oréal's "This Is an Ad for Men" campaign launched in Germany, with clear intentions to go viral. The ad cleverly combines photos of the brand's best-selling lipstick swiveled to rising heights with infographics about how, in general, corporate female leadership boosts company revenue. At the time, L'Oréal, the largest cosmetic company in the world, did not boast a lady-laden leadership; its CEO, Deputy CEO, and CFO were all male. Of its twenty executive heads at the time, only a quarter were women, and only one a woman of color[13]—hardly cause to triumphantly toss one's tube in the air.

Nevertheless, cosmetic companies like L'Oréal were some of the earliest to adopt the language of empowerment to conflate their products—and, by extension, feminine beauty—with feelings of strength, confidence, and agency. The first lipstick campaign credited as adopting femvertising tactics was for Revlon's 1952 Fire and Ice. Authored by advertising maverick Kay Daly, then the highest-paid woman executive in the United States, and photographed by superstar Richard Avedon, the ad presented supermodel Dorian Leigh, then 35, in a tight sequin dress and extravagant red cape-sleeves. Staring at the camera with painted lips seductively parted, Leigh flashes her talon-like nails in front of her face and hip. "For you who love to flirt with fire … who dare to skate on thin ice …," reads the tagline over her waist and thighs. "A lush-and-passionate scarlet … like flaming diamonds dancing on the moon!"

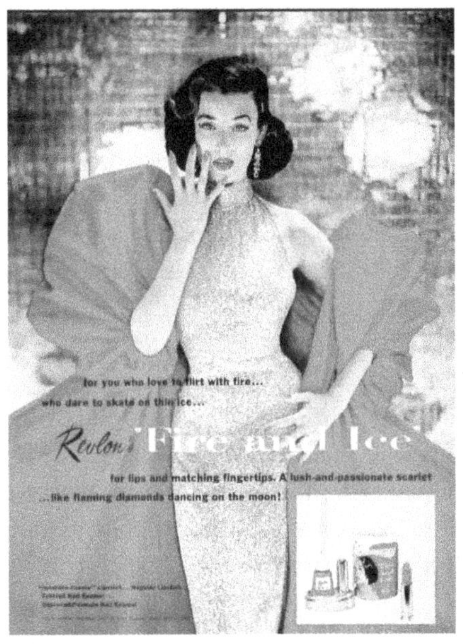

FIGURE 3.1 Revlon's "Fire and Ice" lipstick campaign, 1952.

Much has been made about how no man appears in the photograph, and the woman's sexual desire is abstracted rather than directed at a monogamous partner. But in many iterations of the ad, a quiz appeared on the adjoining page inquiring, "Are You Made for 'Fire and Ice'?" with a list of questions below.[14] Some queries read as proto-feminist ("Would you streak your hair with platinum without consulting your husband?") and others feel downright regressive ("Do you love to look *up* at a man?"). While much of the ad's language celebrates women's sexual desire—and daring—in a time that both were often repressed, the lipstick itself is billed as "a foolproof formula for melting a male."

Still, like all the best femvertising, Fire and Ice made women seem powerful and celebrated their contradictions ("a new American beauty … she's tease and temptress, sire and gamin, dynamic and demure."). While it overtly pandered to nabbing a nebulous male partner, it also summoned a fantasy of a woman whose painted face and glamorous persona were part of flouting, not following, the rules of feminine decorum.

Revlon's campaign anticipated what *Bitch* magazine founder Andi Ziesler terms "marketplace feminism," which includes "you-go-girl tweets and Instagram photos, cheery magazine editorials about dressing to please yourself." As she puts it, rather bleakly, "the fight for gender equality has transmogrified from a collective goal to a consumer brand."[15]

As much personal pleasure as I've taken in the fantasies drummed up by beauty adverts, and believe female pleasure is nothing to knock, I see Ziesler's point. Femvertising can distract from much more worthy goals—especially if the "empowerment" starts and ends with the fleeting pleasure of consumption. Aligned with choice feminism, femvertising encourages women to believe purchasing products is a political act.

Having made all sorts of individual consumer choices that had zero positive impact on gender equality, I reject choice feminism—as I do any consumption-based activism—as a viable course of political action. But I also think that feminine beauty—and not just in cisgender woman—can bring delight to our environmentally and aesthetically imperiled planet.

But What About the Male Gaze???

Twelve years old on my first day at a raucous public middle school, I wore a red tee cinched with a scrunchie over a ruffled, three-tier denim skirt. Also: a trial-size "Plush Red" lipstick I'd purchased for 99 cents. "Nice lipstick! Can I kiss it?" an eighth-grader jeered as I boarded the bus.

I was embarrassed and electrified. A 70-pound, four-foot-something science fair winner who wouldn't grow boobs for another four years, I was unaccustomed to *any* male attention, favorable or not. Was this boy joking? Even a little bit serious? I had no desire to kiss this kid—whose face I never got a good look at—but the outlandish possibility of anyone (even briefly) fantasizing about kissing *me* was admittedly titillating.

In his seminal 1972 book, *Ways of Seeing*, art critic John Berger saw the power (and burden) to attract the gaze as inherently feminine. "Men look at women. Women watch themselves being looked at," he wrote. "This determines not only most relations between men and women but also the relation of women to themselves. The surveyor of woman in herself is male: the surveyed female. Thus she turns herself into an object—and most particularly an object of vision: a sight."[16]

Yikes.

Though Berger rejected gender essentialism—the belief that gender is fixed and biologically determined—to consider the "social presence" of men and women, his thesis on the act of looking has long been taken as dogma when it comes to how men look at women and women see themselves. To dispute the existence of the male gaze feels like a fool's errand; over a century of primarily male-directed cinema confirms its sway, if not its omnipotence. But women look, too—and often at other women.

Can self-adornment lead "the surveyed female" to greater objectification—of herself and other women? Perhaps. But objectification need not equal subjugation: any aestheticizing act inherently leads to an appearance deemed more (or less) pleasing by the arbiters of any given era, and a pleasing appearance need not mean automatic erasure of one's autonomy—especially when millions of women have gained real economic ground over the last half century. I doubt a swipe of Revlon can redact all that.

Even if the male gaze *is* still subconsciously internalized by women today, it is often eclipsed by the gaze of other women, women evaluating and ranking each other, especially online, based on a bevy of enviably rare aesthetic markers. However much it has diversified its ideals in terms of race and ethnicity, the beauty world is hardly a bastion of equality. It never has been and, for all we might aim for egalitarianism, it seems unlikely to ever be so. Lissome bodies, large eyes, and clear complexions continue to dominate; meanwhile, physical assets unheard of during my adolescence—like thigh gaps, glass skin, and "debloated" abs—expand in (often toxic) influence via social media. Lip shape and lip fullness have not been spared such hyper-scrutiny and hierarchization.

Is it likely that girls and women have internalized sexist beauty standards and then exacted them on each other—creating hierarchies informed, if not dictated, by expectations that women be attractive above all else? Certainly. "Pretty privilege" is impossible to extricate from the ongoing legacy of patriarchy. So, too, arguably is any aesthetic choice. In a world where men have for millennia wielded greater cultural and economic power, no choice is 100 percent pure.

But it's also arguably the case that beauty arbiters today—the ones whose opinions on appearances matter the most—aren't even primarily cis, straight men. From Anna Wintour to Bobbi Brown to Kevyn Aucoin to Jeffree Star to Nikki Tutorials, the ones making the rules (whether they're presented as "rules" or not) are almost always straight women, trans women, or gay men. In fact, it's hard to think of one cis, straight man whose opinion really matters in contemporary beauty or fashion discourse today.

Gender Trouble and the Rules of Adornment

What made makeup feel less of an obligation and more a means of creative expression? How might lipstick be a sign of progress, rather than a prop to prop up the patriarchy?

The crudest answer is capitalism: when marketers realized they could sell to women—including to those who do not identify as "feminist"—a more empowering, creative vision of beauty, it worked. Billions of dollars were made by the beauty industry and are no doubt floating about this instant like pastel confetti.

But I think it's also more than that. Call it third- or fourth-wave feminism. Call it liberation from binary constructions of gender. Blame the spate of women who've delayed marriage or motherhood—or choose not to pursue either. After a retrogressive period post-9/11—the scads of Paris Hilton and Lindsay Lohan lookalikes who ruled media—the twenty-first century has witnessed a shift from lip color construed as blandly womanly to something more eclectic and fun. And what Judith Butler called "gender trouble" has something to do with it.[17]

Appearing "girly," or feminine in a youthful way (which, some would say, is a redundancy), no longer means asking to be infantilized. Nor does a colored lip mean that a woman necessarily seeks approval (or sexual attention) from men. Nor, for that matter, does a colored lip mean that a woman *isn't* seeking sexual attention from another woman. (There have *always* been "lipstick lesbians" and gender rebels who've flouted the rules of adornment.)

Butler anticipated this shift in their seminal 1990 book *Gender Trouble: Feminism and the Subversion of Identity*, which advanced the thesis that gender is a *performance* more than anything else. It is not inborn; it is not immutable. "There is no gender identity behind the expressions of gender," they argued. "[I]dentity is performatively constituted by the very 'expression' that are said to be its results."[18] In other words, what is feminine or masculine has less to do with biology as the ability to repeatedly perform certain gestures agreed to fit into either category. Gender troublemakers are those who refuse to follow the script—from androgynous Annie Lennox in 1990 to the trans beauty vloggers who came to transform the vlogosphere in the 2010s.

"Playing a part is an exercise in make-believe," Becca Rothfeld writes in *All Things Are Too Small*, her 2023 apologia for excess, "but this does not mean it is not serious."[19] Referencing Mikhail Bakhtin's theory of the carnivalesque, Rothfeld examines the dual roles of ornamentation and play in all aesthetic ventures. Lipstick, too, can play a part in fashioning a self that finds pleasure in resisting predictability.

Changing one's lip color is possibly the fastest, cheapest route to dramatically changing one's appearance—one reason that many shape-shifting icons (Madonna, Gaga, and Rihanna among them) have embraced wildly varying shades of lip color at crucial intervals in their careers.

There is also sensuous pleasure in the experience of gliding something over the lips on a regular basis, as it involves touching a sensitive part of the body. "Playing" with one's visage can itself be satisfying, even thrilling—perhaps especially when such play bucks gendered or cultural expectations. "Survival does not depend on the exorbitance of art or fashion," Rothfeld declares, "but we are too greedy to settle for survival."[20] In a way, the oft-cited "lipstick effect" during economic recessions—an uptick in lipstick sales when overall disposable income shrinks—is but one example of lipstick enduring as a "necessary luxury" when other indulgences are unaffordable.

Rothfeld concludes that what is unruly and obviously impractical is also at the crux of our deepest erotic selves. Artificial lip shades—colors that flout any fidelity to a prim spectrum of pinks, peaches, reds, and browns that "naturally" appear on the face—defy compulsive femininity precisely because they so loudly deviate from gender norms. What is fake and feminine tacitly reveals that femininity itself is a façade, not something you're "born with" based on a matching pair of chromosomes.

Gaga Feminism

In 2011, I was chosen for a jury in a criminal case. Despite being on the younger side of the group, I was elected "foreman"—in part because, as a writing teacher of nontraditional students, I had experience leading discussions among a motley set of people. Each morning, I headed downtown to the neoclassical courthouse in a glam version of my attire as an adjunct college instructor. I quickly developed something of a reputation, and the security guys who spotted me in line for the metal detector took to calling, "Here comes Gaga," as I approached.

To be sure, I found this hilarious and flattering. I'm of pasty Scots-Irish stock, not Italian, and am older than the pop star. But we both favored heels and sported pale faces. We also wore bright red lipstick.

A few years later, when I experimented with shaggy bangs mid-semester, my first-years started whispering about me during class. "What is it?" I finally asked, suspecting a world map of chalk on my bum. "You look like Taylor," shared a charitable young woman whose name I forget (but, as I do recall, wrote a swell research paper on pit bull regulations). "It's the bangs and the lipstick."

What gender theorist Jack Halberstam dubbed "Gaga feminism" in 2012 has little to do with being mistaken for a celebrity (though I heartily encourage the practice), but rather "a form of political expression that masquerades as naïve nonsense but that actually participates in big and meaningful forms of critique."[21] Lady Gaga represents "both an erotics of the surface and an erotics of flaws and flows."[22] Rather than credit Lady Gaga herself (Stefani Germanotta) as emissary of this "new gender politics," Halberstam sees "some relation in her work between popular culture, feminine style, sound, and motion that hints at evolving forms of sex and gender at a moment when both are in crisis."[23] Rejecting much doctrine of the past, Gaga feminism is "simultaneously ... a celebration of the joining of femininity to artifice and a refusal of the mushy sentimentalism that has been siphoned into the category of womanhood."[24]

And what could contribute more to an "erotics of surface" than lipstick and gloss? Both magnify the mouth, an erotic pleasure center, and announce their artificiality. Like Gaga feminism, lipstick is also about "performances of excess: crazy, unreadable appearances of wild genders; and social experimentation."[25] To Halberstam, Gaga feminists "are not 'becoming women' in the sense of coming to consciousness, they are unbecoming women in every sense."[26]

With his playful twist on "becoming," meaning beautiful, Halberstam envisions a space where, rather than forge feminist solidarity based on biological notions of womanhood, women are realizing that the whole category of womanhood is subject to question. Rather than "become a woman" via menstruation, marriage, or motherhood, one can "unbecome" a woman through embracing artifice. The idea that such a person actively questioning gender is *also* "unbecoming" mocks the idea that, to be beautiful, one has to adhere to prescribed aesthetics.

Accordingly, the art of "going gaga" can be found in "the politics of free falling, wild thinking, and imaginative reinvention best exemplified by children under the age of eight, women over the age of forty-five, and the vast armies of the marginalized, the abandoned, and the unproductive."[27] It's interesting that Halberstam groups "wildness" and "imaginative reinvention" as prominent *both* in young kids and in women past the age considered their aesthetic prime. Rather than doom a woman to obsolescence, female aging is liberating—a way to radically reconceptualize one's appearance rather than stepping in line.

"Going gaga" definitely describes the late Iris Apfel, "the matriarch of maximalism," whose flamboyance made her an icon well into her nineties. Growing old "disgracefully" meant flouting the idea that, the older you get, the less colorful you get to be.[28] Before she passed away at 102, Apfel's boisterous coral-red lip didn't budge. When, at a third of that age, I was compared to her by a twenty-something Brooklyn barista, I took it as compliment *way* more flattering than any likeness to Taylor or Gaga. (I also tagged Apfel in a tweet that said as much, which she *hearted* … swoon!)

"[W]e can use the world of Gaga to think about what has changed and what remains the same," Halberstam writes, "what sounds different and what is all too familiar, and we can go deep into the question of new femininities."[29]

Of course, Gaga, the living human, has never lived in a "postcapitalist world" and, once being a monster became less profitable, swapped gender spectacle for more recognizable modes of womanly performance—from dipsomaniac-civilizing in *A Star Is Born* (2018) to gold-digging in *House of Gucci* (2021).[30] Germanotta wasn't going to squander her glorious monstrosity on actual revolution. Not when there was money to be made from starring in Oscar bait and launching her own cosmetics line.

But that doesn't mean the "question of new femininities" has to "die with a smile," as one Gaga hit goes. Black women and other women of color have been reinventing femininity for years. And it's only relatively recently that white women—feminists included—have opened their eyes to see that.

SIDEBAR #2: THE MYTH OF THE RED-LIPPED SUFFRAGETTE

Google "red lipstick" and "suffrage," and pages of links will spill from a number of credible outlets, all recounting—and usually extolling—the penchant among First Wave American feminists for a lacquered pout. Most of these modern-day news sources reference the May 4th. 1912, suffrage rally in Manhattan, when some 15,000 women marched from Washington Square to Carnegie Hall. It's a pretty, and pretty provocative, picture: women in white dresses and white parasols storming Fifth Avenue on a spring day, their chanting mouths an urgent red.

And it's almost certainly a total lie—and not a white one.

One book asserted Elizabeth Cady Stanton, Charlotte Perkins Gilman, and "other notable feminists" all attended the rally in "painted lips as a badge of emancipation."[1] But

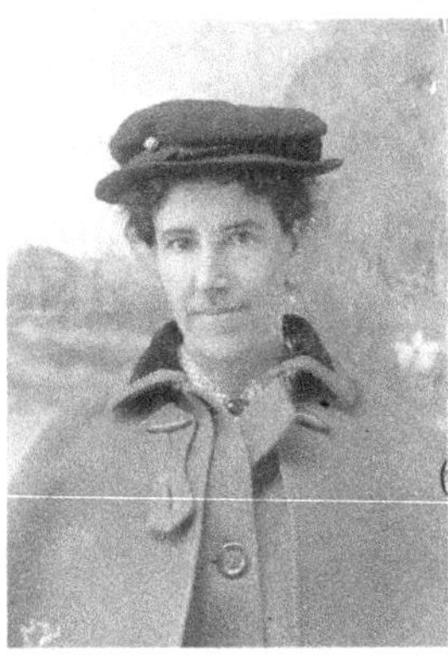

FIGURE 3.2 Charlotte Perkins Gilman, 1899. Harvard University, Schlesinger Library on the History of Women in America.

Stanton had passed away a decade earlier, and try as I might, I have failed to locate one photograph of Gilman appearing in lip color of any kind (though she does look chic in a newsboy cap).[2] As historian Lucy Jane Santos has recently noted of the May 1912 suffrage march, "there was a great deal of interest in what the women were wearing by the press and a great deal of planning by the organizers." In other words, were women boasting crimson mouths, it would have been written about in the press at the time. Santos explains, "Whilst the reports may have varied on how successful the march was in terms of rallying people to their cause, there is one thing that all of them have in common. Absolutely no mention of lipstick, red or otherwise."[3]

How would such a myth proliferate? Blame Elizabeth Arden. Not Elizabeth Arden the person—otherwise known as Florence Graham, pioneer of American beauty culture—but Elizabeth Arden the powerhouse *brand* that has circulated the myth.

What we do know is that, in 1912, Graham joined the New York rally, shocking staff at her 5th Avenue boutique.[4] Having previously scoffed at feminist gusto, the enterprising Welsh-Canadian businesswoman likely saw the suffrage movement as a sure way to rub shoulders with the white, educated, Protestant elite, a group which she was both desperate to infiltrate and cater to in her tony skincare "salons." As Santos points out, Graham's 5th Avenue flagship store had only been open two years at the time of the 1912 suffrage march, and even though "cosmetic use had gained in popularity and acceptability in Europe … it was very much not a thing in New York."[5]

About a century later, as femvertising came to dominate the beauty industry, twentieth-century revisionism followed suit. What better way to encourage women to embrace a brand—or a lipstick shade—than to link it to a right that virtually *all* Western women cherish, whether or not they call themselves feminists? After all, if you're already apt to feel powerful wearing red lipstick, how much *more* powerful will you feel if you reckon yourself a suffragist who brazenly took to the streets?

While this fantasy is seductive, it obscures the much more complicated history of lipstick, feminism, and the so-called "lipstick feminism" of the late twentieth century. Revisionism infuses the past with today's fashionable ideology. It can also hold the past to unfair scrutiny among those who already know how everything turned out.

Was Elizabeth Arden an ardent feminist? No. Did she give out red lipstick to the masses? Almost certainly not. Has this legend made the brand a lot of money? Unquestionably.

In 2019, the brand dredged up its supposed suffrage legacy for its "March On" campaign. A limited-edition lipstick ("signed" in red by spokeswoman Reese Witherspoon) was sold globally to benefit women's rights. "Moved by our founder, a woman dedicated to empowering women," the ad declares, "we are donating 100% of the proceeds to UN Women. Join us as we march on to empower women everywhere. Wear the lipstick as a sign of solidarity."

Solidarity with whom, exactly? Visiting the webpage of UN Women,[6] I found a host of striking female faces from across the world—from Sierra Leone, Sudan, Afghanistan, and Gaza. Some are young, some are old; some are smiling, some are somber. None, however, are wearing visible lipstick.

Lest I seem to finger-wag at *all* femvertising, I am not. If one feels powerful wearing red lipstick (as do I!), go for it. But the founder of Elizabeth Arden wasn't looking to "empower" women so much as climb the social ranks and become fabulously rich. (Which, to her credit, she did.) When the words "march" and "solidarity" are directly linked to her legacy, her self-serving ambition is conflated

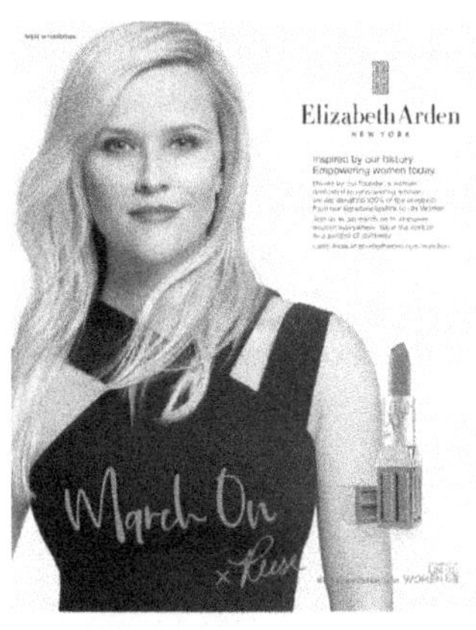

FIGURE 3.3 Reese Witherspoon in Elizabeth Arden "March On" campaign, 2019.

with the goals of actual feminists who risked jail time and even their lives for the cause of suffrage. Sorry, Reese, that's not the same.

But, just as it's best to avoid revising the past to pull a profit, it's best to resist judging historic actors by today's ethical standards. I don't judge Florence Graham for cynically glomming on to the suffrage movement, any more than I judge my late grandmother for smoking while pregnant with each of her nine children. I also don't see the point in turning every successful woman in history into a bona fide feminist or conflate something like lipstick with a cause as noble as voting rights. Given that women in other countries *do* wear lipstick as an act of resistance today, suggesting that American feminists did so in 1912 conflates their wildly different cultural contexts, and blurs one's sense of what constitutes public dissidence.

An object like lipstick can be rich with meaning, even political implications, without itself being a revolutionary tool. Overstating the case only warps our vision of where we came from—and where we are today.

Handwritten Excerpt #3: Shaela, Younger Millennial

When I was a kid, I would stand in front of a mirror with a ketchup packet saved from my McDonald's Happy Meal, carefully recreating the iconic lipstick scene from the Disney Movie The Little Mermaid. It's the one where Ursula is peak sea witch villian - doing her hair and makeup like a boss right before belting out a catchy number about poor, unfortunate souls. She picks up a sea creature in a shell, squeezes it, and deftly rubs its blood (?!?) on her lips to stain them a perfect shade of red. I was obsessed.

When I was a kid, I remember multiple occasions where I would stand in front of a mirror with a ketchup packet saved from my McDonald's Happy Meal (a rare treat), carefully recreating the iconic lipstick scene from the Disney movie *The Little Mermaid*. It's the one where Ursula is peak sea witch villain—doing her hair and makeup like a boss right before belting out a catchy number about poor, unfortunate souls. She picks up a sea creature in a shell, squeezes it, and deftly rubs its blood (?!?) on her lips to stain them a perfect shade of red. I was obsessed.

4 WHITEWASHED BEAUTY, APPROPRIATION, AND LIPSTICK LEGACIES

Marilyn Monroe flashes naked teeth between slick cherry lips. Dita Von Teese channels goth burlesque with a pert carmine smirk. Taylor Swift swoons over a mic in Pat McGrath's MatteTrance, and the shade sells out in seconds.

Flip through your mental Rolodex (or Insta feed) of lipstick icons, and several are likely white women. The "French Girl" look, emulated by American celebs like Kendall Jenner and Lily Collins, pairs minimal eye and face makeup with a red lips on a (presumably) pale face (never mind the fact that French girls are a range of complexions). As a white woman, I've not once been told that a bright lip contradicted my racial identity. From the Brothers Grimm to the Body Shop, I've been taught since girlhood that a bold mouth against alabaster skin makes for a pleasing mien (not to mention, pleasing men). Snow White herself was described as boasting "lips red as blood and a face as white as snow." As a kid with dark hair and Charmin complexion, I admittedly appreciated resembling at least one classic Disney princess. But the white-as-snow bit also felt suspect, conflating so-called innocence (which I patently lacked) with genetic features beyond one's control.

Meanwhile, Black women and girls have been discouraged from wearing certain lipsticks for at least a century, taught that red doesn't flatter dark skin or that bold hues connote sexual promiscuity.[1] Latinx women have similarly been discouraged, lest they seem "saucy, exotic, loud, sexual, and sometimes even tacky."[2] Like most double standards based on race and class, those surrounding lipstick have hardly disappeared, even as white supremacist beauty ideals have loosened their grip on mass culture.

When my middle-school teacher, Mrs. Tayborn, who was Black, singled me out for my too-red lips in 1992, were race and class at play? As I recall, *she* wore lipstick in middle age (and looked damn good). She was also employed by the St. Louis Public School District, underpaid and overworked decades before I pedaled my white frame and bright lips into her social studies classroom. If *she* had ever been discouraged from donning red lipstick for fear that it would attract the wrong attention—and for professional Black women those rules have always been more stringent—she may have been trying to protect me, a most studious student, from naively sending out the wrong impression.

Or maybe my firetruck mouth was distracting the woman from her lesson on the Spanish-American War. Who knows?

Inclusion and diversity specialist Chloe Benson notes that "American beauty discourses often reproduce the dominant white worldview which privileges white femininity as the ideal; this standard of white beauty is reproduced in subtle and inferential ways within the cosmetics industry."[3] Many people of color who *do* wish to wear bright lipstick have found that most brands just don't show up on darker lips. Seema, 40, shared with me her mother's penchant for Estee Lauder's "Maple Sugar" lipstick: "Back in the '90s, it was one of the only colors that looked good on Indian skin, as so much of the makeup available was made for white people."

Similarly, MAC's "Ruby Woo"—a cool red launched in 1999, that has graced the lips of Rihanna and Tracy Ellis Ross—has been long known as a staple for women with darker complexions.[4] Mariama, a Black, queer "elder Millennial" I surveyed, listed MAC's "Heroine" as her all-time favorite lip shade. "Beauty companies have done a poor job at providing a variety of shades for deeper skin tones," she stressed, "which fuels this false conception of certain colors being off-limits."

Eighteen years after "Ruby Woo"'s debut, the wild success of Fenty Beauty, the cosmetic line Rihanna founded in 2017, catalyzed what beauty insiders have dubbed "the Fenty Effect": major brands both high and low paying attention to the millions of women with darker skin tones.[5] "Say what you will about Fenty as a corporation," Mariama told me, "but it truly changed the game for Black women and people of color who love beauty products—pushing other companies to be more inclusive and innovative in their shade ranges."

Take Pound Cake, for example. Vexed that most lip colors didn't work for her Black skin, in 2022 Camille Bell founded the delectably named cosmetic line, launching five shades of red liquid lipstick that, at $24 a pop, sold out in minutes.[6] A decade prior, ex-Wall Streeter Melissa Butler whipped up a series of highly pigmented vegan lipsticks in her Brooklyn kitchen. After her pitch for "The Lip Bar" was panned on Shark Tank in 2015, viewers crashed the website with 30,000-plus hits.[7]

Watching Butler and her creative director Roscoe Spears pitch to Shark Tank today is physically uncomfortable in its epic cringe: two young Black women—donning electric violet and cerulean lips, respectively—in front of three middle-aged white men, one Black man, and one middle-aged white woman, all who reject not only their product, but the appeal of their adventurously colored lips.[8] Judge Kevin O'Leary jokes that Spears "looks like she needs to be resuscitated"; he later calls the two women "colorful cockroaches." That same judge declares, "The chances that this is a business are practically zero." The sole Black judge tells them, "You are never going to create anything new in this world—it's lipstick."

Guess who got the last laugh? Over the next two weeks, approximately 120,000 people visited The Lip Bar's website,

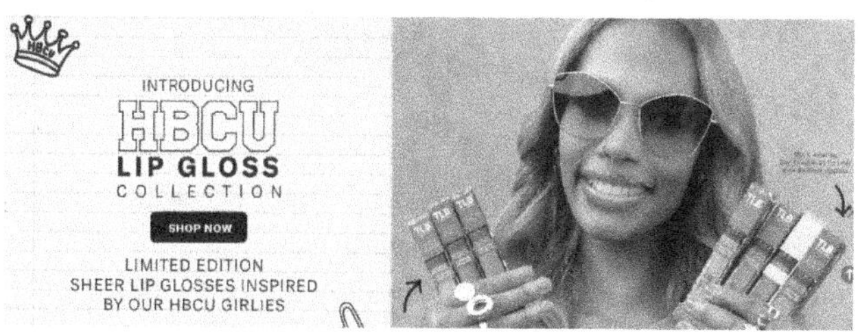

FIGURE 4.1 The Lip Bar Website, HBCU Lip Gloss Collection, featuring Melissa Butler, 2024.

definitively establishing a target audience.[9] In 2017, Butler opened her flagship store in downtown Detroit. To date, the brand is carried in over 2,000 brick- and-mortar stores, including CVS, Walmart, Target, and Meijer, as well as online—and, at $13.99, is relatively affordable. In 2024, The Lip Bar debuted its HBCU lip gloss collection, inspired by the makeup trends at historically Black colleges and universities, of which Butler herself is a proud alum.

Will lip gloss—or any consumer product—put an end to racist beauty standards? Of course not. But Butler and Bell, and others like them, are proving that many lipstick lovers—across race and gender—prefer an eye-popping teal to a prim pink any day of the week. They are also proving, as women of color have done for centuries, that beauty ideals evolve with more diverse participants in beauty culture.

Whitewashed Beauty Standards

American studies scholar Kristin Denise Rowe has noted that, while "dark skin, kinky hair textures, large lips, large round noses, and large/curvy bodies are often denigrated …mainstream beauty standards have socio-historically privileged these corporeal features most closely linked to whiteness."[10]

Given that, to my knowledge, puny lips have *never* been applauded—"thin-lipped," after all, is an epithet connoting malevolence or disapproval—the fact that full lips have been racially disparaged throws into relief the bald hypocrisy of white supremacist beauty ideals. On a white woman, full lips are a boon, a presumed sign of youth and fertility; on a nonwhite woman, *too-full* lips become, like anything else "extra,"[11] *too* erotic, *too* showy, *too* much.

In the early twentieth century, when exaggeratedly large lips were common to racist caricatures and a staple of Blackface minstrelsy, many Black women were cautioned against calling attention to their mouths at all. "Whether it is popular or not," a Black newspaper beauty columnist cautioned her readers in 1930, "a person with large lips should be very careful when wielding the lipstick. Remember that you are making your mouth more prominent and use your judgment as to whether you can afford to have more prominent lips."[12]

Nearly a century later, Kennedy, 24 and "a light-skinned Black woman," confided to me: "I personally find pretty much every color unflattering compared to my lips' natural shade. Perhaps it has to do with the fraught history of depictions of Black women's lips as oversized and bright red."

Mariama shared with me that her "greatest pet peeve is when Black women are told, or have internalized, that they shouldn't wear bright or bold lipsticks because it accentuates the fullness of our lips in 'negative' ways." She ardently stressed, "There is nothing more beautiful or sexy than a Black woman rocking a bold, bright lip color." Ola, a Caribbean-British ESL instructor in her late thirties, shared that she admires lipstick on Black women specifically. "It showcases our lips' size, shape, and diversity," she attested. "Lipstick enhances our natural beauty and gives confidence."

But as with much of racism and sexism, the internalized variety can manifest most vehemently. Women can be just as likely as men, if not more, to openly patrol other women's beauty habits. Treasure, 53, described to me the shade thrown her way when her daughter "took up the habit of wearing a very bold red lip" in third grade. "Within the context of Black parenting norms, my parenting style is very permissive," she explained. "But I distinctly remember holding her hand walking down the hallway and into the lunch room. There were some older Black women who gave me judgmental looks. For my part, I was much more interested in protecting my daughter's self-esteem and bodily autonomy."

Louisa, 45, a London opera singer and nail technician of Ghanaian descent, wears red lipstick most days, but recalls pushback for it in her teens. "My birth mother remarked that the shade of red, which was scarlet, didn't suit me," she recounted. "She had the hubris to liken me to a prostitute for wearing it."

Likening lipstick to sex work, of course, goes back millennia. In the early twentieth century, when lipstick consumption was on the rise in the United States and the United Kingdom, the "association between cosmetics and prostitution alienated Black women from the beauty industry," writes historian Melissa L. Baird, "as drawing attention to their sexuality was the very thing they sought to avoid." What complicated matters was that the beauty industry was also one of precious few places in which enterprising women could be upwardly mobile. "Black beauty culture developed … as a form of political contestation, a source of pleasure, a practice of self-making, and the basis of livelihoods," writes sociologist Maxine Leeds Craig, pointing out that "the Black-owned Overton Hygiene Company was among the first manufacturers to develop facial cosmetics specifically for Black women."[13]

Arguably even more than white working-class entrepreneurs like Florence Graham (aka "Elizabeth Arden"), Black women have been eager to seize opportunities to thrive economically *within* the beauty industry. The ascent of Black-owned businesses in the late nineteenth century can be tied in part to the industrialization of effective hair-straighteners, which proved extremely profitable; their rise can also be connected to the assumption that grooming could impart a sense of dignity that would uplift the race. Madam C. J. Walker, America's first Black millionaire, built her empire on the presumption that "pride in race should involve pride in appearances." The extent to which such pride was based on stamping out signs of Blackness has been subject to debate, though it's clear that Walker herself didn't see hair-straightening that way.[14] As Leeds Craig asserts, "though disparaging images of Blacks, and Eurocentric beauty standards, pervaded popular culture and undoubtedly influenced the way many African Americans saw themselves, media images never entirely defined Black aesthetics."

But to look "respectable" in the twentieth century often meant downplaying anything that could be interpreted as sexualizing, putting Black women in a Catch-22 when it came to makeup, especially lipstick. "Although American definitions of beauty excluded Black women," writes Baird, "the consumption and production of beauty products based on these ideals offered Black women social and economic benefits that were hard to ignore."[15]

Predictably, when a marginalized group of people has been sexualized, pleasure from self-adornment can prove much more fraught. But that doesn't mean Black women eschewed the beauty industry. For many Black women of the twentieth century—and today—unequal access to the same range of products, and the expressive potential therein, was but one of many instances of inequality to be redressed.

"Black Is Beautiful" and Lipstick Dissonance

Not unlike femvertising adopting (and diluting) feminist rhetoric to push products to consumers, by the late 1960s, "Black Is Beautiful" was not only a political slogan, but a marketing tool to sell a bevy of cosmetics to Black women. Avon, with its history of Black sales reps, was among the leaders in this respect, placing a series of ads in *Ebony* magazine proclaiming lip color and a natural Afro as complementary.[16]

A new
kind of world
happening
all around you
Patterns by Avon
AVON
COSMETICS

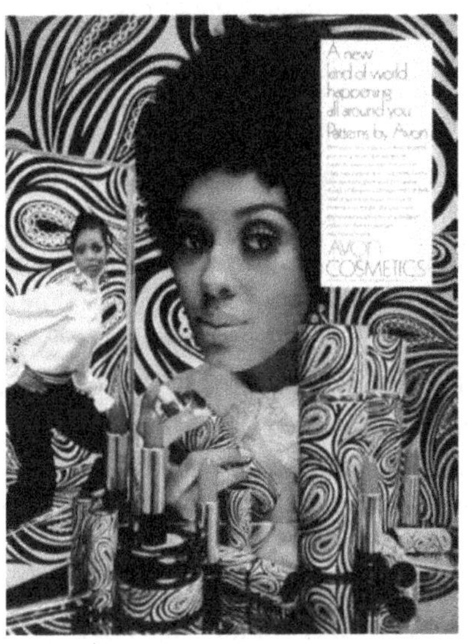

FIGURE 4.2 Avon lipstick ad in *Ebony* magazine, late 1960s.

"I love to try out different colors. It's the only way to buy makeup."

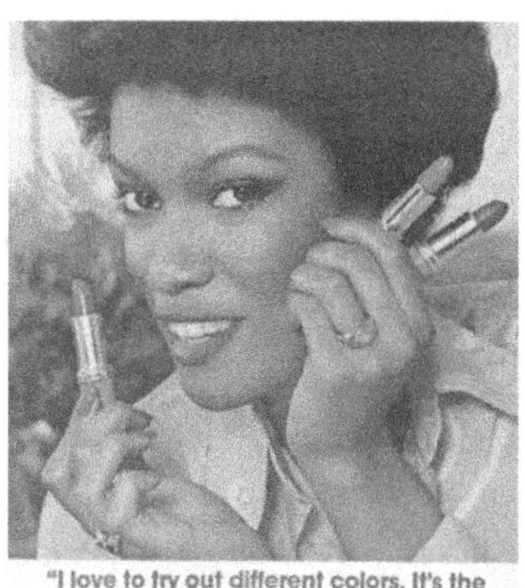

FIGURE 4.3 Avon lipstick ad in *Ebony* magazine, late 1960s.

"As 'Black Is Beautiful' expanded beauty standards to include dark-skinned black women," writes Baird, "new cosmetics companies flooded in to market products to meet the newly modified standard."[17] Of course, not everyone was thrilled with the tenets of "Black Is Beautiful" at the service of white-owned—or even Black-owned—cosmetic companies. Whether it was Avon and Revlon, owned by whites, or Fashion Fair and Posner, both Black-owned companies, the imperative to paint one's face *in order to be beautiful* was hardly a revolutionary credo.

Revlon wedded to ethnic pride? Consumption conflated with liberation? It didn't take a trip to the Fashion Fair counter for Black women to realize something was *up*. As Baird put it, "While Black women were more represented in beauty ideals, they still were not liberated from them."[18]

In her 1995 essay "Beauty Laid Bare: Aesthetics in the Ordinary," radical feminist bell hooks makes the case that feminine aesthetic pleasure, while crucial to well-being, was not the same as excess consumption. For Black women who "have been increasingly socialized by the mass media ... to assimilate into the mainstream," she argues, "[h]edonistic consumerism is offered as a replacement for healing and life-sustaining beauty." By contrast, "[l]earning to see and appreciate the presence of beauty is an act of resistance in a culture of domination that recognizes the production of a pervasive feeling of lack, both material and spiritual, as a useful colonizing strategy."

In other words, beauty itself—as seen in oneself and in others—is vitally important. But its pursuit is not synonymous with how much you splurge on Sephora or the local beauty supply store. (A lesson clearly germane to those of *any* race!)

African American women who came of age in the late twentieth century were exposed to a wide array of Black lipstick icons whose beauty didn't conform to white dominant culture. Tiffany, 52, points to androgynous icon Grace Jones as lipstick inspo. "Their features were so striking, and the entire look screamed, 'I'm running this. I'm fabulous and people are paying me for it.'"

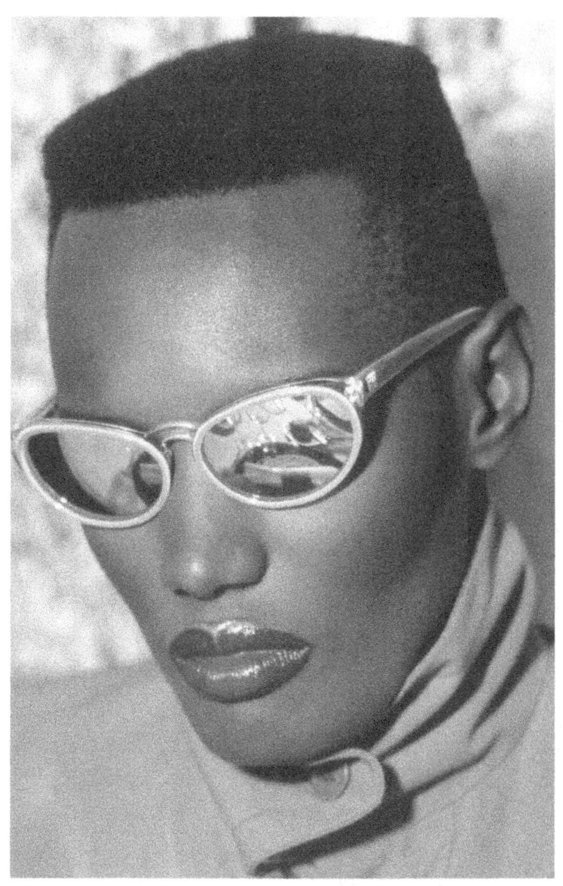

FIGURE 4.4 Jamaican singer Grace Jones posing for a photoshoot. Italy, 1981. Photo by Angelo Deligio/Mondadori Portfolio via Getty Images. Credit: Mondadori Portfolio / Contributor.

Maurice—a self-described "Black fat transfemme Millennial"—cited "Black women in the '90s" as the ultimate lipstick influencers. "The overlining, the way they did ombre lips before it was a thing," she shared, "everything about the makeup look for Black girls in the '90s, the soft glam, speaks to me."

Mariama, who also grew up in the 1990s, embraces the idea of lip color as a shield of adornment. "Lipstick can be affirming for women who wish to wear it," she underscored. "I don't wear lipstick for men or for anyone else. I wear it for me—I smear it on like armor, like a protection spell that will keep me bold, and curious, and fiercely true to myself."

"Armored in Beauty"

Marcela, a 48-year-old Tejana novelist, first wore lipstick for a fourth-grade *escaramuza*, an equestrian event which consists of eight-woman teams riding horses in synchronized maneuvers. A typical *escaramuza* costume includes a bright red lipstick to complement one's *charro* hat and ruffled skirt. "There's so much about *escaramuza* that is so feminine, but it's such a strong and athletic sport," she informed me. "You're literally dressed to the nines in a Victorian-era costume with your face all made up, but you're negotiating choreographed moves while you control a thousand-pound animal!"

Citing Mexican singers María Félix and Selena Quintanilla-Pérez as two women whose lipstick she admires, Marcela prefers "matte red with blue undertones" as her choice shade. "I wear it because I feel good when I look good," she elaborated. "Sometimes if I have a hard day, I especially need to feel armored in beauty."

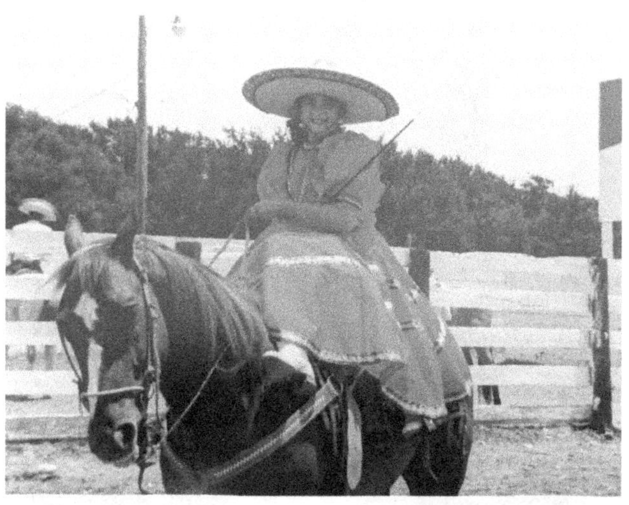

FIGURE 4.5 Marcela, age 10, wearing lipstick for *escaramuza* debut.

But lipstick stigmas can also deter certain Latina women from donning brighter shades. "A red lip on a white woman tends to be perceived as elegant, timeless, and classic,"

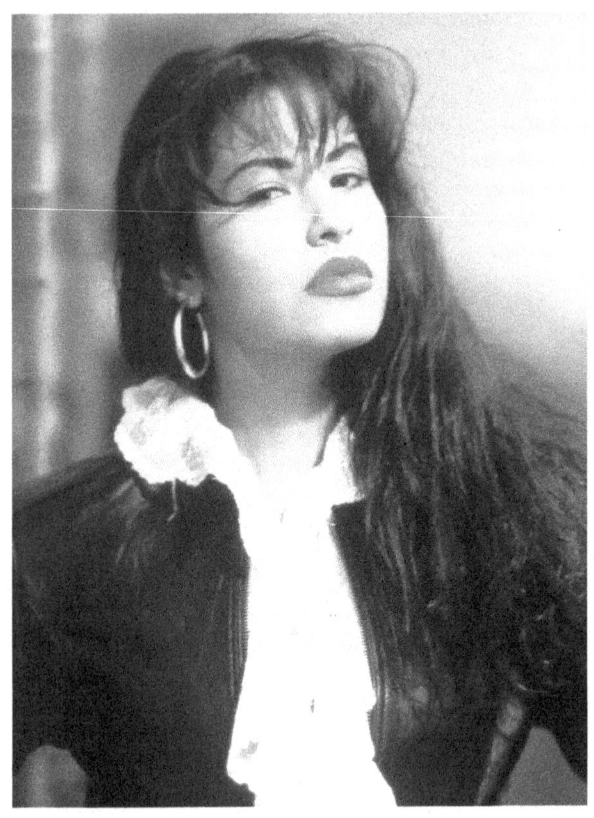

FIGURE 4.6 Pop star Selena Quintanilla-Pérez, 1992.

Regina Merson, founder of cosmetics brand Reina Rebelde, told the beauty blog *Thirteen Lune*. "Yet, for some reason a red lip on a Latina is perceived totally different … we already take up all the air in the room, so how dare we call attention to our voices and our appearance so overtly."[19]

Alexandria Ocasio-Cortez is perhaps one of the most famous, and famously outspoken, Latina lipstick lovers. "Any attempt to make my femininity trivial or unimportant is an attempt to take away my power," the Congresswoman asserted in an interview with *Elle* magazine. "So I'm going to wear the red lipstick."[20]

With few exceptions—America Ferrera comes to mind—Western media tends to celebrate a fairly Eurocentric vision of Latina beauty: light-skinned and narrow-nosed, but with a curvaceous physique. Sociologist Mónica G. Moreno Figueroa has explored the ways in which Latin America's history of forced racial mixing of "indigenous peoples, African enslaved people and European settlers," otherwise known as *mestizaje*, still privileges those of lighter complexion.[21] To women subject to these competing cultural aesthetics, lipstick may be one of the least fraught facets of their beauty routine.

For those who are biracial, lipstick can serve as a reminder that beauty habits often carry latent ethnic relevance. Kaylei, 21, who is half-Latina, recalls her *Titi* Carmen, a "Puerto Rican ball of fire" who frequently visited her Milwaukee childhood home. "Titi wouldn't dare leave the house without a full face of makeup," Kaylei recalled. "Her favorite was a smooth, burnt red lipstick. On her, the warm maroons and deep browns looked classy and natural. She let me try her lipstick once, but I looked like a clown. It was a reminder that I only look like one half of my heritage."

Bharatanatyam and South Asian Lipstick

South Asian women boast their own lipstick traditions that have nothing to do with Taylor, Madonna, or any other Western imperialist export. Chief among them would be the popularity of red lip color. "In South Asia, red has always been in," writes Ayesha Le Breton, "from vermillion to bridal outfits, from Preity Zinta's dress in *Kal Ho Naa Ho* to the rage of *Bulbbul*, from Durga's sari to Kali's tongue, from Rajput attire to vocalization marks in Qurans."[22]

Smitha, who is 25, pansexual, and of South Indian descent, relayed to me how she first started wearing lipstick at age five when performing *Bharatanatyam*, the most popular form of Indian dance, traditionally performed by a woman on a bare stage.[23] "Lip color is symbolic and has a beautiful meaning in South Indian classical dance," she shared. "It is celebrated as an aspect of femininity, strength, and performance." In addition to elaborate costume and jewelry, heavily kohled eyes, and darkened eyebrows, red lipstick is standard—the red connoting the fortune and joy associated with Hindu marriages.[24]

Growing up with a "positive view of lip color," Smitha was surprised to witness the "slut-shaming" of girls wearing lip color at her suburban middle school, "depriving people's choice of how they want to express themselves." To my surprise, Smitha viewed lipstick on women *of any race* as an opportunity to be stigmatized—by men and women. "When I see Congresswoman Ocasio-Cortez, Taylor Swift, or other powerful women wear bright red lipstick, I have a 1% reaction of 'Oh God, they are coming to attack her,'" she explained. "By 'they,' I mean misogyny, patriarchy, and haters! People are truly intimidated by women who make their presence seen, especially when they take back the power of the meaning of lip color."

Young women of color today are apt to vocally challenge white supremacist assumptions of beauty ideals and how they pertain to intersectional identities. As Safa, who is trans, 28, and of South Indian descent, put it, "Contrary to the stereotypes about Muslim women, there is much less anxiety about the aesthetics of the body than found in Protestant and Catholic communities. Because women are usually spending their most intimate time with other women, not as a rule but as an affinity, there is a more playful relationship to the male viewer."

"It's not uncommon," Safa signed off, "to see a beautiful queer Muslim woman rocking a hijab with a bold lip."

Injectables, Lip Kits, and Instagram Face

When Lydia, who is white and working-class, was growing up in Oregon in the 1990s, she was teased for "having big lips," and chose more subdued lip colors to deter attention. But thirty years later, she shared with me that "it can be fun to flaunt them now that full lips seem to be considered attractive."

What accounts for this voluptuous swing in opinion? "Instagram Face." As Jia Tolentino explored in her 2019 *New Yorker* exposé, the collusion of social media, Facetune, and plastic surgery in the 2010s, gave rise to a "beauty ideal that favored white women capable of manufacturing a look of rootless exoticism." Named for its ubiquity on the photo-sharing app, "Instagram Face" approximates a cyborgean form of femininity. "It has catlike eyes and long, cartoonish lashes; it has a small, neat nose and full, lush lips," writes Tolentino. "The face is distinctly white but ambiguously ethnic—it suggests a National Geographic composite illustrating what Americans will look like in 2050 …."[25]

In other words, by imitating traits less common to Caucasians, white women retain the benefits of racial privilege and benefit *from* looking subtly "exotic." What does that mean for lipstick? It means that, for many, the *color* of one's lips has become less important than their *volume*.

In the United States, surgical lip augmentation has grown 60 percent since 2000; in 2021, the market was worth $1.9

billion, and is expected to grow over seven percent by 2030.[26] In a UK Snapchat poll of men and women between thirteen and twenty-four, over half of some 51,000 respondents said they viewed procedures like lip fillers "as comparable to getting a haircut or manicure."[27] As Tolentino attests, "Thanks to injectables, cosmetic procedures are no longer just for people who want huge changes, or who are deep in battle with the aging process—they're for Millennials, or even, in rarer cases, members of Gen Z."

While these fillers produce a fuller pout via injectable hyaluronic acid, the effect often feels ethnically appropriative: the feature historically maligned on a Black person is mimicked by a white one. Unsurprisingly, in a 2017 survey of Americans, sixty percent of Black respondents indicated that they are "generally against the procedure," the highest rate of disapproval for any racial group.[28]

Cultural theorist Meredith Jones posits the rise of the Kardashians, Kim specifically, as abetting this lippy appropriation. "Over the years, we have seen the Kardashians play with racial hybridity and adopt Black embodiments including hairstyles, fuller lips, and larger butts," she writes. "This is cultural appropriation and is sometimes referred to as 'blackfishing.'"[29] One of the crown jewels of the Kardashian empire, Kylie Jenner's non-surgical "lip kits" overtly vow to mimic the effects of injectables. When they launched in 2015, these kits sold out in less than ten minutes online, and they remain popular a decade on. Around the same time, a viral trend called the "Kylie Jenner Lip Challenge" encouraged young white women to suck into a shot glass to temporarily achieve the volume for which Jenner was celebrated.

What's the difference between painting one's mouth for illusory fullness versus plumping one's lips via syringe? Like all injectables, lip filler has a host of potential side effects—from bleeding and bruising to asymmetry, all irrelevant to lipstick on its own. Filler is also a lot more expensive—the average cost in the United States hovers just under a thousand dollars,[30] and that number can swell faster than your plush pucker if you live in a posher region. But for me, at least, the crucial difference is that an injectable, while hardly permanent (it dissolves in about a year), reinforces the *ideal* of permanent, "naturally" full feminine lips. Lipstick is more upfront about its temporary and artificial nature.

But rather than finger-wag specifically at filler aficionados, I consider this latest trend as another unfortunate example of how fickle—and racialized—feminine beauty standards have always been. Personally, I'd rather fake a cupid's bow with a bright color than look naturally bee-stung, no matter the beauty hive mind of the moment.

Lipstick Legacies

In "Black Girls Don't Wear Red Lipstick," a 2024 exhibition at the Austin Central Library, photographer Leta Harrison openly called out lipstick stigmas with 42 portraits of African American women in a wide array of crimson shades.

Affectionately cribbing the exhibit's title from a lecture given by multi-disciplinary artist Kam Franklin Harrison is the first Black woman photographer to headline the library's gallery, and sees the show as "a love letter to the boldness of Black women."[31]

"I remember my ex telling me I looked like a clown when I started wearing red lipstick," Leta told me. "I almost stopped wearing it because I was not as confident back then, and his words stuck. Glad I didn't listen!"

For so many women of color whose self-image developed in the early twenty-first century, rejecting mandates about "respectable" self-presentation has become an essential part of forging an identity less fettered by white beauty ideals. Of those I surveyed about lipstick, a greater percentage of women of color cited their mothers or grandmothers as imparting the value of adornment as a source of dignity and pride—suggesting that perhaps, for those racially marginalized by the beauty industry, lipstick legacies *within* one's own community have left the most indelible (kiss) print.

"I bought a tube of Maple Sugar recently," shared Seema. "My mother died fifteen years ago, and it's a nice reminder of her … like traveling back in time, inhabiting the shoes of the generation of women who came before me." Claire grew up in Port-au-Prince, Haiti, and also counts her late mother, Germaine, as a lipstick icon. "I always remember her wearing deep red color lipstick," she explained. "I loved how it made her look radiant, classy, elegant, and powerful. I loved how it highlighted the contour of her lips and brought out her facial features."

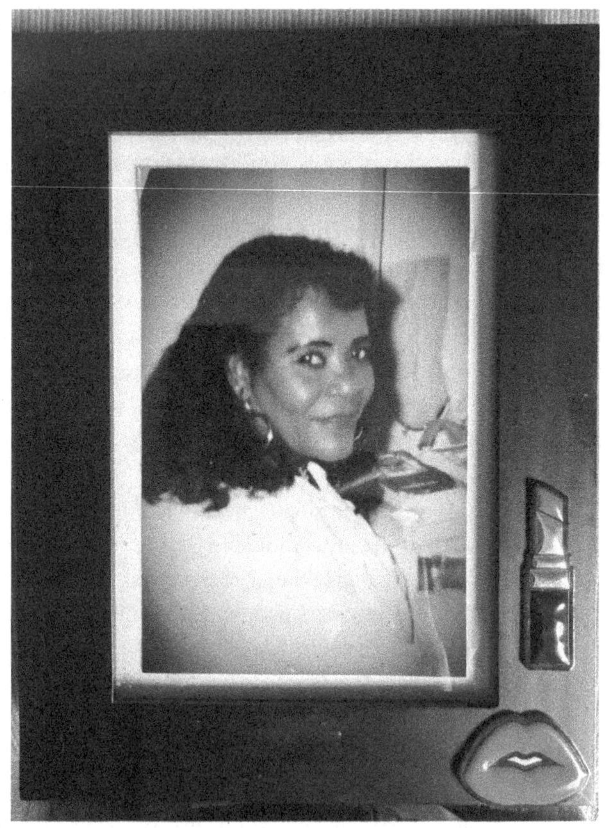

FIGURE 4.7 Portrait of Germaine in lipstick frame.

Dorris, 40, identifies as nonbinary and does not wear lip color, but vividly detailed their first lipstick memory in relation to their single mom. "I am sure I used her lipstick, probably getting ready for Easter service," they told me. "I would also accompany my mom to the Fashion Fair makeup counter at Dillards. Back in those days, Fashion Fair was really the only makeup company that catered to Black women, and it was owned by the Johnson family, who also owned *Ebony* magazine. While she could have bought her lipstick anywhere, I assumed that brand loyalty played a role in her buying it at Fashion Fair."

Others recounted the magic of witnessing their mothers get ready as a child. "I used to sneak in my parents' bathroom all the time and play with my mom's eyeshadow and lipstick," relayed Sheenu, 43 and a Christian first-gen Indian American. "I was fascinated by the colors, smell, textures, packaging, brushes. It seemed fancy and expensive to me as a kid." Ella, who is 19, half-Chinese and half-white, recalled childhood mornings spent "sitting on my mom's bathroom countertop" as she prepared to go to work. "Just before leaving, she'd pick her lipstick color out of the top drawer, apply it, and then lift me off the counter to kiss me goodbye," she recounted. "I remember thinking how beautiful she looked, and how her lipstick made her look so grown-up. I couldn't wait for the day I could choose a shade from her drawer and wear it myself."

For Davon, 37, a Black trans genderfluid femme who teaches dance and drag performance, trying on their grandmother's lipstick was both transgressive and affirming. "Being conditioned as a binary male, I felt it was 'wrong' to play with her makeup," they explained, "but I felt such a pull to try them on. I can remember seeing women on TV dramatically applying lipstick and I wanted to replicate those scenes. So I did! In the secrecy and privacy of my grandmother's bedroom."

Mariama's memory of her Grandma Ana, "smoking Camels in her kitchen, a ring of maroon lipstick staining the end of the cigarette as she ashed," speaks to how powerfully the visual, tactile, and olfactory coalesce in our tenderest memories. "The same rough soft hands that once bathed me in the sink now engaged in a graceful dance of indulgence," Mariama reminisced. "*Inhale, exhale, ash, inhale, exhale, ash.* Her lips left stains and prayers all around us."

SIDEBAR #3: FOUR DECADES OF LIPSTICK LYRICS AND MUSIC VIDEOS

"I nail my mouth to the evil taste of lipstick, inhale the scent of someone else's lipstick . . ."

Wadded up Kleenex smudged red. A can of aerosol deodorant. A tube of lipstick tossed onto a scatter of counter clutter. After a two-second shot of cosmetic detritus, Suzi Quatro struts onscreen, clapping her hands to the beat of the drummer behind her. Her lips are a neutral dusty mauve, her bass guitar a lustrous red. "I'm tired of making up while you've been making out with someone else's makeup," she spits in her signature punk parlando.

It's 1981 and Quatro, a pint-sized, leather-clad, four-string-plucking badass, may be the first to feature lipstick in a music video.[1] "Lipstick" confronts a common twentieth century trope: catching (or in this case, *tasting*) male infidelity through the tell-all lipstick stain. While Quatro clearly isn't against wearing makeup—her eyes rimmed with smoldering charcoal as she scowls at the camera—lipstick is a way to distinguish herself from her lover's lesser side chick, a woman whose lipstick is described as "sticky," "scarlet," and "purple," before dismissed by Quatro as "trashy trashy trashy" in the song's snarling send-off.

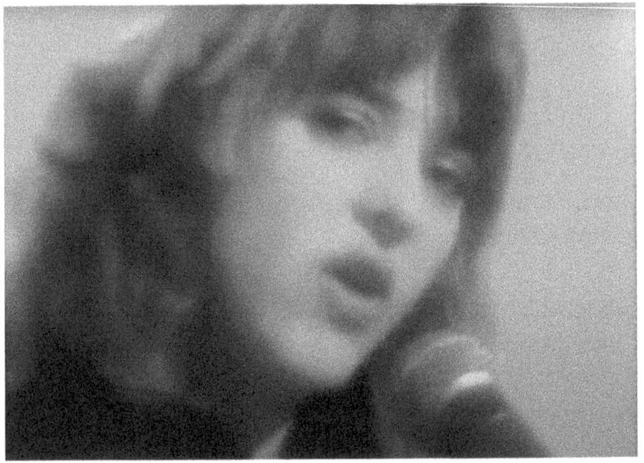

FIGURE 4.8 Suzi Quatro, "Lipstick" music video, 1981.

As a totem of romantic competition, feminine seduction, patriarchal repression, and erotic lust, lipstick has swiveled its head into a range of music videos since the multimedia genre's explosion in the 1980s. Tracing lipstick's ruddy arc across the years, we can see how wildly its meanings diverge. Conspicuous lip color can, after all, signify a million things—from class status to sardonic camp.

In 1994, Tori Amos's US video for her piano anthem "Cornflake Girl" presents a coven of quarreling young women driven through the desert in the back of a pickup truck.[2] Upon the track's climactic bridge, the quartet-plus-Tori circle a beefcake cowboy bathing in a metal trough, disarming "the man with the golden gun" by synchronously cocking their lipsticks as though from invisible holsters at their hips. As each pink or mauve bullet juts out from its metal tube, the effect is comically phallic and femme at the same time. In the brutal terrain of female cliques, beauty remains a potent, if unreliable, weapon—one which Amos, her grin a glistening pink, wryly acknowledges and critiques.

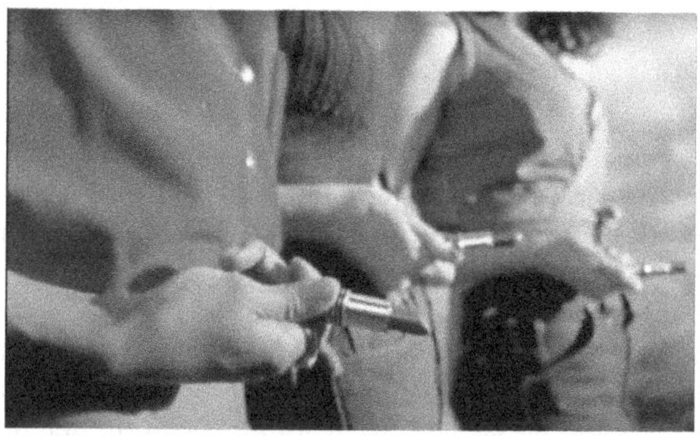

FIGURE 4.9 Tori Amos, "Cornflake Girl" music video, featuring Revlon lipstick tubes, 1994.

A year later, the alternative rock band Eve's Plum, fronted by Colleen Fitzpatrick, conflated wearing lipstick with female voicelessness. "My lipstick was glue stick," she sings in "Lipstuck," "it sealed my fate, not even able to communicate."[3] Vaguely grunge in vibe, the track overtly recalls Second Wave feminism's suspicion of feminine adornment. "I've been a victim of fashion, unjustly applying berry passion," goes the final refrain. In a song where vanity means being a "slave to makeup," appearing willfully feminine might as well mean handing over your free will. But by 2000, in her later solo turn as pop act "Vitamin C," Fitzpatrick would not only drop her anti-lipstick stance but lend her moniker to a lipstick shade by Tommy Hilfiger.[4] This was around the time that anti-feminine feminism faded into Third Wave reassessments of girly adornment. By the early aughts, erstwhile edgy rock stars like Courtney Love and Nina Gordon swapped their torn fishnets and rumpled slip dresses for French manicures and blown out coifs. Pretty was undeniably *in* again, and often so anodyne that even lipstick lovers like myself longed for the days of an angsty anti-makeup manifesto.

Over two decades later, pop-cultural attitudes toward lipstick—and overtly femininized self-adornment—have veered again, as evidenced by distinctly queer iterations of hyper-femme aesthetics. Take nonbinary icon Janelle Monáe's 2023 music video for "Lipstick Lover," an ode to sapphic eroticism set at a bacchanalian pool party where booty cheeks vie with painted pouts for the artist's, and the viewer's, visual attention.[5]

“I like lipstick on my neck,” Monáe declares, as an array of puckered-up femmes approach her supine form. “Hands around my waist, so you know what’s comin’ next.” If lipstick in the mid-1990s was capitulation to patriarchal, and presumably heterosexual norms, here it is both a badge of Black, queer, feminine approval and a mark of messy, sticky pleasure—as well as a stand-in for *other* lips playfully mimicked across the video. “Leave a sticky hickey in a place I won’t forget,” Monáe begs. “Baby, I’m obsessed, get me undressed.”

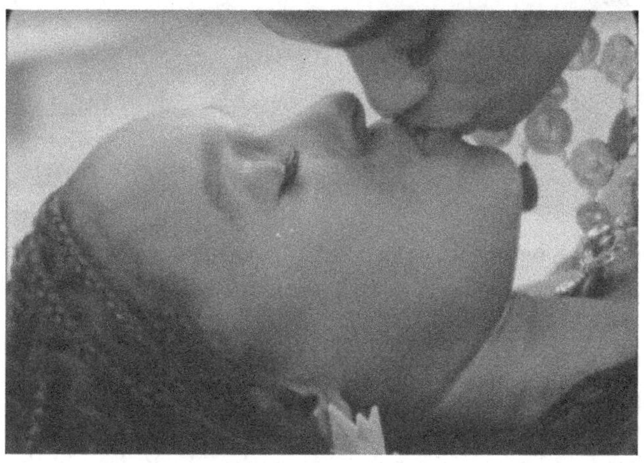

FIGURE 4.10 Janelle Monáe, “Lipstick Lover” music video, 2023.

Queer desire, femininity, and lipstick form an intrepid triptych in the form of pop star Chappell Roan, whose

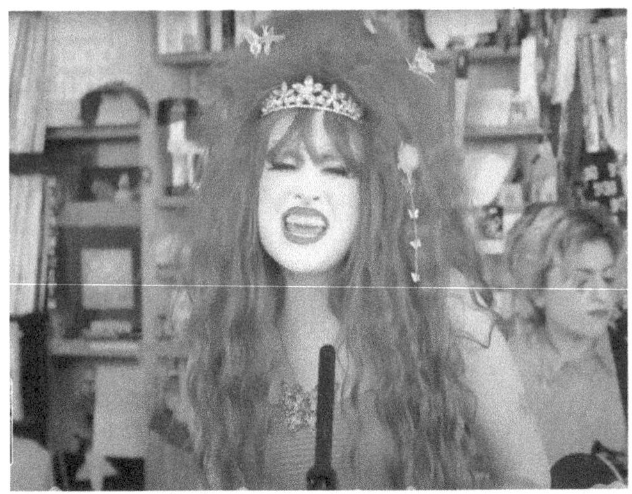

FIGURE 4.11 Chappell Roan, NPR "Tiny Desk Concert," 2024.

persona betrays both her rural Missouri provenance and the glittery legacy of drag performance. In her 2024 Tiny Desk Concert for NPR, Roan is surrounded by seven femme musicians, each wearing red lipstick, blue eyeshadow, a pink button-down or a red party dress.[6] Roan's fiery hair is piled in a foot-high bouffant above a rhinestone tiara, her face layered in kabuki-like powder. "Knee-deep in the passenger seat and you're eating me out," she croons to an inferably female auditor, her lipstick displayed on not only her cupid's bow but prominently on her two front teeth. "But we're casual now, we're casual now." Calling attention to hook-up culture's endurance among Gen Z, Roan recasts hyper-femininity in a lesbian context. Camp vulnerability and country vibes mingle in a mashup of queer exuberance and Marie Antoinette libertinism: between songs, Roan waves a pink feather fan.

Sterling Tull, the makeup artist and drag queen responsible for Roan's "camp-meets-couture" look, has emphasized since that lipstick on the teeth was wholly intentional, as the singer wished the band to look like they "went through hell, they just cried their eyes out, they just had enough of it and smeared their lipstick." These chaotic touches "add to Chappell's look, because Chappell has a few things that are kind of going awry on her face."[7] Roan's lipstick gone "awry" on her teeth brings a camp sensibility to both mock and celebrate feminine performance that resists traditional heteronormative constructs. As Tull puts it, her lipstick "embolden[s] people to become more interested in drag and playing with their identity and gender."

From Suzi Quatro's "trashy trashy" lipsticked nemesis to the "white trash" splendor of Chappell Roan, showy lip color has gone from being a telltale sign of hetero canoodling to a sign of the humiliation of falling for a woman who refuses to return your texts. Bright lipstick isn't just for the heartbreaker; it's also for the heartbroken. Clearly, lipstick is no longer limited to straight girls trying to steal someone's shitty boyfriend.

Handwritten Excerpt #4: Dorothea, Gen Z

The goth pop artist Allie X is a lipstick and fashion idol to me. Her look is vamp, classic, weird, and seamless; she draws on 80s new wave, contemporary drag, classic Hollywood, and horror. I admire her ferocity - she's not afraid to push to the extremes of a look, to venture into high glam and/or the uncanny, or to experiment. I saw her in London in the summer of 2024; she wore a sort of deconstructed wedding dress, and her lips were the color of crushed blackberries. She's adaptable, chimerical, and individual.

The goth pop artist Allie X is a lipstick and fashion idol to me. Her look is vamp, classic, weird, and seamless; she draws on '80s new wave, contemporary drag, classic Hollywood, and horror. I admire her ferocity—she's not afraid to push to the extremes of a look, to venture into high glam and/or the uncanny, or to experiment. I saw her in London in the summer of 2024; she wore a sort of deconstructed wedding dress, and her lips were the color of crushed blackberries. She's adaptable, chimerical, and individual.

5 A FEMME-FRIENDLIER FUTURE?

"Yes, I took a full chomp out of the bundle of lipstick."
—Chappell Roan[1]

Around 2019, something started changing—both at the university where I teach and in broader popular culture. Feminist undergrads defended corsets in their analysis essays. "Bimbo feminism" blossomed on TikTok,[2] with influencers vying to fight the patriarchy in pink bodycon and false eyelashes. One student of mine surmised that I had a "fashion designer girlfriend" because I "wear bright lipstick and artistic clothes." Male first-years sported fingernail polish, and not just those aiming to attract other men. Several of my friends and colleagues came out as nonbinary, of whom several maintained a playfully feminine style accented by quirky earrings and shimmery lips. At least a few students adopted "they/them" pronouns, which did not necessarily mean they projected an androgynous look.

The frilly accoutrements censured by, if not banished by, from feminist circles at my college about twenty years ago no longer seem (as) at odds with feminist ideology. Anecdotally, among those under thirty-five, a feminine look need not suggest conservative politics, cisgender female heterosexuality, or even adherence to conventional gendered demeanor.

My rebellious rejection of sartorial staidness has started feeling a lot less … rebellious.

All of which is to say: most of the bright lipstick I see these days isn't on women looking to lasso a Chad. Nor is it on female service workers looking to keep their jobs. It's on transfemme baristas, beauty vloggers with neck tattoos, and—wait for it!—college professors who weren't informed, as I was in the late '1990s, that academic success requires the defenestration of heeled footwear and lurid lip gloss.

During the pandemic, a younger colleague of mine, who wears a matte red lip daily, joined a Facebook group for faculty interested in dramatic makeup techniques. "The point of the group was to push the boundaries of what you can wear on your face and still command respect," she told me. These days, irreverence for institutional authority can mean *wearing* noticeable makeup, rather than shunning it.

I can already hear the naysayers snarking that these lipstick-loving women and nonbinary folks aren't evidence of it being any less oppressive, but rather evidence that we are dupes of femvertising, tricked into believing that wearing beauty products is a virtuous form of "self care." As already acknowledged: I don't disagree! At least not entirely. But I also don't think the synthesis of feminism and femininity can be exclusively tied to advertising. As female students predominate in American higher ed, at both the undergraduate and graduate levels, could it be that *looking feminine* no longer means looking less capable? That lipstick no longer overtly declares, "I'm assiduously aiming to attract a man, a man who will, *à la* Calgon, 'take me away' to a more economically secure and socially sanctioned place ...?"

A lot of lipstick lovers aren't at all concerned with luring the male gaze. Millennial journalist and broadcaster Alex Berg defends her bright lipstick as *part of* her queer identity, rather than its antithesis. "I derive power from lipstick when I wear it as an adornment that does not serve straight desires," she wrote for *Them* magazine, "a kind of power that exists beyond amplifying femininity for the sake of being seen as worthy of attention from straight cis men."[3]

Feminine identity can also blithely co-exist with other visual and physical signifiers traditionally read as masculine, even manly. A former student of mine, Kaylei, highlighted US Olympic rugby player Ilona Maher as a lipstick icon. "Her femininity seemed to be viewed as a novelty among female athletes, which struck me as odd because some Olympic athletes, like gymnasts, nearly always have a sparkly eye or lipstick/gloss to draw attention," Kaylei explained. "But it was the first time I've seen makeup in the Olympics in a 'less feminine' sport like rugby."

Maher, who is 28, sees bright lipstick as transgressive, not capitulatory. "I play a sport that is traditionally very masculine. You have to be, supposedly, very manly to play," Maher told *Allure* magazine. "So I wear makeup [on the pitch] to give a big 'eff you' to having to sacrifice my femininity. Even while I wear lipstick or have mascara on, I can still tackle hard, run hard, and be a great rugby player."[4]

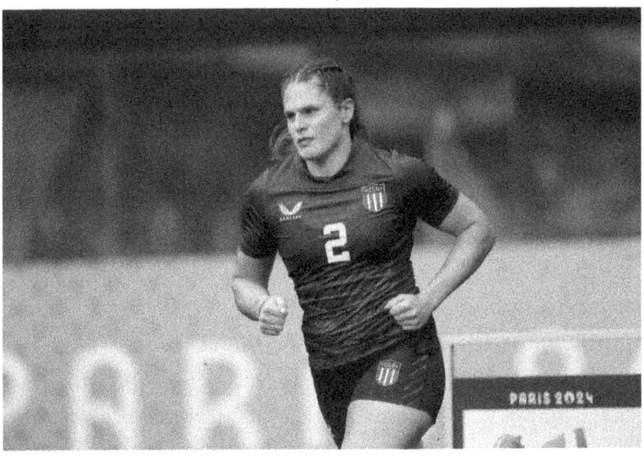

FIGURE 5.1 Ilona Maher in the 2024 Summer Olympics, Paris.

Some Gen Z women I interviewed expressed that they're inspired when men wear lipstick, too. Sydney, 20, shared, "A lot of my guy friends wear lip products and look great, and their use of the product is helpful to the female community because it separates our specific identity from makeup, making it more of a unisex way to express yourself."

How many women today feel the need to actually *wear* lipstick on a regular basis? Not many. In a YouGov survey from 2023, only 10 percent of American women 18–29 wore makeup daily, compared to nineteen percent of those 30–44, 21 percent of women 45–64, and 24 percent of women 65 and up. But that doesn't mean that younger women eschew makeup entirely, or lipstick specifically. Women 18–29 were the *most* likely to wear makeup "a few times a week," and the *least* likely of any age to "never wear it." By contrast, a full 36 percent of women 45–64 reported that they never wear it, as did a solid 26 percent of those 65 and up. The most popular forms of makeup for women in all age groups were lipstick and mascara—the two products that arguably make the biggest impact with the least effort.[5]

Obviously, this is just one survey and should not be overinterpreted.[6] But it seems pretty clear that makeup, including lipstick, is more polarizing for older women than it is for younger women; otherwise, why would so many more women over thirty wear it everyday *and* so many more women over thirty choose not to wear it at all? If anything, Gen Z women seem to embrace makeup, but on their own terms. Interestingly, women who identified as Democrats or Biden voters were *more* likely to wear lipstick than their Republican or Trump-supporting counterparts, suggesting that the choice to paint one's mouth is about more than accepting or rejecting conservative views on gender.

In my own survey of women and nonbinary people between 18 and 29, most indicated that they wear lipstick sometimes, but not as a matter of course. Meredyth, 19, "will occasionally wear lipstick or lip gloss if … going out." Livia, 28, mostly wears "tinted balms." Elizabeth, 28, shared, "I rarely wear makeup of any kind, and I don't wear lipstick/tint/color at all." Smitha, 25, "wear[s] ChapStick or hydrating lip balm" on a daily basis, but added, "[on] days when I feel like dressing up—whether to go out to Target or head to the office or for dinner—I enjoy matching my lip color to my outfit!" Sarah, 28, "wear[s] lipstick about once a week—for Date Nights, Girls Nights, or when [she's] wearing contacts." Bridget, 28, wrote, "I do not wear lipstick/gloss much in my everyday life, but I do wear it when I am performing in dance or theater, or if going out or dressing nice." Like many Gen Z and Millennial women, she expressed that bright red lipstick "seemed to be too 'much,'" even though she saw its aesthetic appeal.

Kaylei, 21, was among the few to "wear some form of lip product everyday," her favorite product "a tinted, plumping gloss." Her reasons? "I feel *wrong* without it. It makes me feel powerful, classy, and the slightest bit sexy." Angela, 18, had a similar response: "Lip color transforms me into a better version of myself—at least it does in some sort of psychological way. I feel as if all my best traits have been enhanced." For Angela, the creative aspect of lipstick is a major appeal. "I love the way I can mix colors together to match my outfits," she shared. "Having a bunch of colors at my fingertips makes mixing different colors so much easier and I love experimenting with different looks. For example, I had a specific mix of colors for my performances for speech and debate and a completely different color for my debate rounds."

For young transwomen, lipstick's expressive potential can be complicated. Dorothea, 24, confided that she has "a slightly occult, trepidatious relationship with it," as she is "early on in her transition." She elaborated: "While I admire it on others, and love the artistry of it, I worry that it looks 'artificial' on me personally, that it calls more attention to an area of my face I'm not quite the most comfortable with yet. Of course, this entirely has to do with my own dysphoria." Dorothea referenced Imogen Binnie's 2013 cult classic *Nevada*, "in which the protagonist, a transwoman, cautions against bold lip makeup as it draws attention to the jaw and the upper lip." But Dorothea has also "recently started using a buildable lip stain, to experiment with varying levels of pigmentation depending on comfort—from just a tint during the everyday to bolder for special events and parties." For some transwomen, wearing a bright, bold color can be the mark of claiming their own feminine identity. "I always found the dark red lip so iconic, and a staple of my favorite film stars," Dorothea shared, "so I would like to eventually get to the place where I feel comfortable doing so!"

"Clean Girl" and "Natural" Beauty

An aversion to wearing daily lipstick among younger women may well be related to the indomitable rise of the "Clean Girl" on TikTok and Instagram over the past five years, an aesthetic that valorizes skin "clean" of vivid color, blemishes, or even pores. Predictably, most prominent "Clean Girl" influencers like Hailey Bieber are thin white women whose salient assets include preternaturally high cheekbones and symmetrical features, features often (ironically!) enhanced through plastic surgery. In other words, the "Clean Girl" look is hardly achievable for the average woman, and its ostensibly "natural" ideal often encourages even *more* consumption of beauty products. The goal isn't actually to *be* natural so much as to dupe everyone that you are—bravo!—effortlessly radiant.

While peddling platitudes like "real beauty is within," Clean Girls visually push the opposite idea: that real beauty is surface-level, a sign of racial privilege and genetic fortune more than any other factor. The idea that being "naturally" beautiful in a feminine way is the same as being "clean" further endows genetic inheritance with disturbing virtue: by Clean Girl logic, unnatural feminine beauty—or a lack of beauty entirely—might as well mean you rolled your physical and spiritual self in the mud. One's character is as soiled as her visage.

All of this feels a bit … Victorian. No matter her quasi-progressive rhetoric, the Clean Girl is a conservative throwback to panic over lipstick and sex work. She also reinforces the illusion that femininity itself *is* natural and that "natural" is morally superior. Remind you of an earlier chapter? That's right: the "Clean Girl" is a priggish twenty-first-century version of Puritanical white feminism.

The "Feminine" Fallacy

"Would you mind taking off your lipstick?" How many times have I heard this before a tumble in the hay (or, more likely, a white-sheeted bed or eggshell loveseat). Like a lot of what counts as "feminine"—not least period blood—lipstick inevitably stains. But, arguably more than any other beauty tool, lipstick is said to anchor an alluring, feminine look.

As to whether bright lipstick actually attracts men or turns them away, the answer is just as messy. Anecdotally, some men have been worried about stains or have found the taste off-putting; still others might take it as a sign that I am "high maintenance" (ironic given how easy it is to put on lipstick versus subtler beauty enhancers). Women's media has, time and again, reinforced the notion that men prefer the "natural look," which is essentially the same as saying that (surprise!) men seek out women who are conventionally beautiful based on genetic munificence.

"Science Shows Men Like Women with Less Makeup," declared *Time* magazine in 2014,[7] as though to shock its female readership. About a decade ago, one scholarly study found that twenty-year-old straight men prefer *less* makeup than women applied to themselves for a night out; (presumably straight) women also preferred less made-up female faces, at least when looking at photos of other women.[8] Lo and behold, beauty and pop psychology forums took this conclusion and ran with it.

What would have been more precise? "Really Young Men Like Really Young Women with *Some* Apparent Makeup, But Not Loads of It (At Least Not So Much that One Can Immediately Perceive the Excess in a Photograph)." Also more accurate: "Really Young Men React Negatively to Intense Makeup, Regardless of How Much of It Is Actually On."

The reason I stress the stark difference between *intensity* of makeup and the actual *amount* applied should be obvious to anyone who's aspired to the "natural look": it is often more laborious and demands a lot of products. "Natural" makeup—such as barely there lip color and facial highlighter—is often more expensive and takes just as long, if not longer, to apply. For many women, cis and trans, presenting as naturally feminine is, in a way, *less* natural than just looking overtly made-up.

In response to the online frenzy over the "scientific" news about the male aversion to cosmetics, British journalist Martha Mills tweeted a pic of herself (in her words) resembling "a freshly washed potato" sans cosmetics next to a selfie where she wears "natural looking makeup." Shocking absolutely no one who has ever worn makeup, the Straight Lads of Twitter overwhelmingly preferred the "barely there" look—comprised of twelve separate types of makeup, lipstick but one of them.[9] Did these men have any clue that the "natural look" took so much work (and money)? Doubtful.

It's no surprise that straight guys might spurn a conspicuously painted face for all sorts of reasons—not least the assumption that somehow their *own masculinity* is more intact if they prefer a face that looks "naturally" feminine. Given how many men have, historically and today, been attracted to transwomen (often not realizing it),[10] the reification of "natural femininity" seems a safeguard against the mercuriality of the male libido, and the flurry of homophobic and transphobic anxieties stirred up as a result.

There is nothing "natural" about masculinity or femininity that need be shielded from the dangers—and delights—of artifice. In the animal world, male creatures tend to be the flashy ones, from fire-finned guppies to azure-crowned fairy wrens. Since our rise to the top of the food chain, the proclivity to self-adorn has also been "natural" to human beings. The modern predilection to cleave artifice from nature, specifically regarding femininity, has more to do with sex panic than anything else.

If shunning makeup makes someone feel more comfortable with their appearance and identity, I'm all for it. But resorting to the naturalistic fallacy, that an unadorned face is *morally better*, both conflates nature with virtue (questionable at best!) and ignores the prevalence of artifice in the so-called wild. Appearing "naturally" feminine simply reinforces the idea that femininity itself is a natural resource tied to those with specific hormones and genitalia, when of course it is really a cultural construct with ideals that careen back and forth within varying eras.

When men tell me that I look "prettier when I wear less makeup," it doesn't make me feel better about myself; it makes me wonder if they lack the artistic capacity to appreciate how creatively I make up my face. I'm also not much for appearing "pretty." Forget the pleasant and picturesque. I'd rather look—and be—sublime.

And as far as "natural" beauty, I'd prefer to look a little fake. It feels a lot more honest.

A New Age of Feminine Influence

James Charles. Nikki De Jager. Jeffree Star. Born in 1999, 1994, and 1985, respectively, these three content creators boast a total of 55 million followers on YouTube alone, 54 million on TikTok. As of early 2025, their videos have been Liked nearly 2 billion times. Among beauty-forward women under forty, these three are about as famous as Cindy Crawford, Linda Evangelista, or Christy Turlington were to a Gen Xer in 1990.

What do Charles, De Jager, and Star have in common? All of them don artfully imagined, chromatically varied, and expertly applied makeup, and all encourage their followers to do the same. All of them identify as queer (Charles and Star are gay men; De Jager, known as "NikkiTutorials," came out as trans in 2020). None of them are cisgender women.

If Clean Girls represent one popular aesthetic for Millennials and Gen Z, gender-nonconforming beauty gurus are their vibrant flipside. I started hearing of these influencers about a decade ago whenever one of my (usually straight female or gay male) students wanted to write about them. Having never scrolled beauty vlogs myself, I realized their mass popularity when I spotted Morphe x Jeffree Star products at my local Ulta Beauty store around 2020. Jeffree Star Cosmetics, his own brand launched six years earlier, is reputed to be worth over a billion dollars.[11]

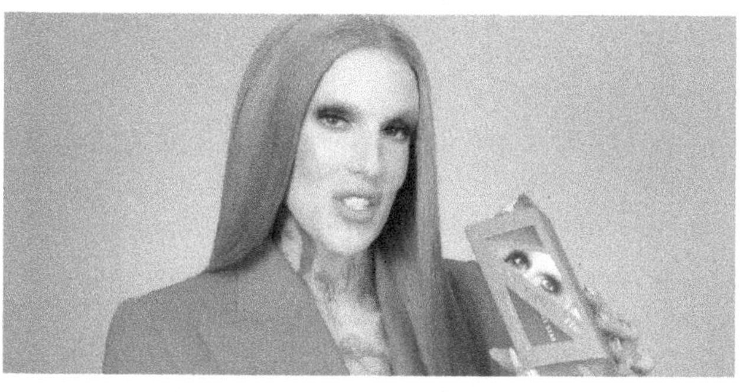

FIGURE 5.2 Jeffree Star's "Jeffree Star x Morphe Brushes Reveal," YouTube video, 2020.

James Charles's line, Painted, which launched in 2023, has had a bumpy beginning beyond the purview of this book. In terms of visual marketing, Painted seems a spin-off of Lady Gaga's Haus Labs, merging racial diversity and gender-nonconformity with vibrant cosmetics. The "Master Paint Bundle," comprising fourteen shades of "ultra pigmented, long lasting paint that can be used a million different ways in your makeup routine," is, at this writing, sold out despite its $195 price tag.

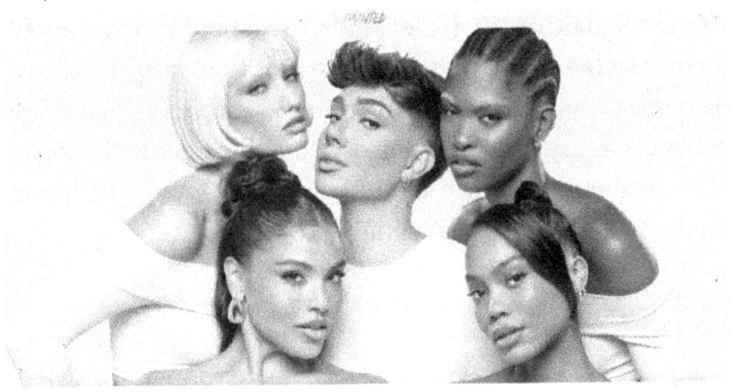

FIGURE 5.3 Painted Website, James Charles at Center, 2025).

In her 2020 volume *Made-Up: A True Story of Beauty Culture Under Late Capitalism*, Quebecois author Daphné B. references Jeffree Star and James Charles as freely as she does twentieth-century philosophers like Kathy Acker, bell hooks, and Roland Barthes. Like a lot of women her age (30 at the time of the book's publication), Daphné feels at once bewitched by beauty content creators and repulsed by the ravages of capitalism. What makes digital beauty culture so addictive, she argues, isn't the perfection of its stars, but rather the vulnerability of their onscreen personae. "We want to see the cracks," she proclaims. "We want chipped vases we can identify with."[12]

Paradoxically, beauty influencers like Star, Charles, and De Jager (along with ciswomen like Jaclyn Hill and Tati Westbrook) are as *flawed* as they are flawlessly made up. They must be "real" to sell themselves, but that performed realness is, by definition, unstable. "[I]f authenticity is perennially in danger of becoming compromised," Daphné writes, "if it's forever under the microscope, it's because in accusing someone of inauthenticity, we're also reinforcing the idea that its inverse—the authentic—genuinely does exist, that there really is a beautiful, true, and pure YouTube channel somewhere in the world."[13]

Of course, this "pure" world is as chimeric as any vision of beauty. No matter their inevitable cancellation for inauthenticity, or worse—both Star and Charles have been accused of some hefty misdeeds—influencers thrive off the fickle nature of online appetites. And these days, a taste for beauty feels more variegated than ever. "Today's digital beauty culture is much more inclusive than the one I remember from my childhood," writes Daphné. "Beauty is no longer too young, too skinny, too white—now it's Black, it has acne, it's fat, disabled, and wrinkled, it comes in all genders and all ages."[14]

While she may overstate her case—beauty culture is still awash with thin, white, cishet women—the fact that millions of women, men, and nonbinary folks are inspired by gender-nonconforming beauty gurus is just one more reason that lipstick today feels less fettered by traditional gender roles. And if, as Daphné argues, vulnerability is what it takes to seem authentic these days, that cuts across gender lines. Counterintuitively, makeup can be a way to declare oneself authentic: "I have flaws," it declares, "but I'm happy to colorfully distract you from them."

Have Your Lipstick and Eat It Too ...

The meteoric ascendance of hyper-femme, queer popstar Chappell Roan late 2023 is just further proof of a new era of lipstick consumption. And by consumption, that also means the literal variety. In a photo shoot for *Interview* magazine in 2024, Chappell takes a bite out of a duct-taped wheel of sixteen red, pink, and coral lipsticks, the lower half of her powdered face smeared in wax.

Born Kayleigh Rose Amstutz in Willard, Missouri, a three-hour drive southwest from where I was born almost two decades earlier, Chappell appeals to the millions out there with a hunger for feminine dazzle *and* progressive gender attitudes. That she herself is from one of the reddest

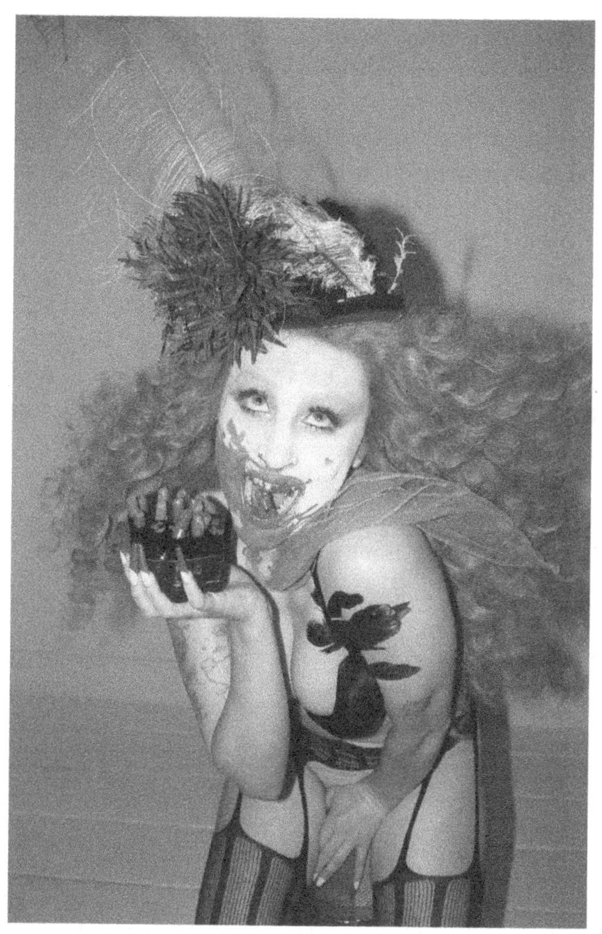

FIGURE 5.4 Chappell Roan, *Interview* magazine, 2024. Photo Richie Shazam.

parts of the United States merely reinforces what may seem, to some, an inherent contradiction. Rather than reject her flyover roots, she embraces the joy in their tacky connotations. She—and her legion of "Pink Pony" fans—turn classical femininity on its classist head, all while remaining consistently vulnerable in her lyrical content (her title of her debut album *The Rise and Fall of a Midwestern Princess* is but one example).

For those raised during a time in which lipstick signified capitulation to the male gaze, a throwback to compulsory heterosexuality, and a symbol of blithe self-objectification, Chappell might befuddle more than embolden. But her mainstream fame doesn't seem to be temporary. For my part, I welcome her as a sign that, despite enduring sexism, racism, classism, transphobia, and heteronormativity, feminine power can emerge from a gloriously varied spectrum of visual possibilities.

Gothic-Pixie-Glam Girl (at Any Given Age)

This snowy Saturday afternoon, I head out to the nearest suburb and purchase The Lip Bar's Nonstop Liquid Lipstick at Target. Dubbed "Drama Queen," it is the darkest shade I have worn in years: a velvet matte black with violet undertones. After applying it in the restroom, I stomp through rock-salt puddles in the parking lot to scout out my hatchback behind a mountain of ploughed snow. As I catch a glimpse of myself in the windshield of a passing truck, the banal task becomes baroque: I am no longer a shopper lost in a maze of SUVs, but a winter warrior with skin and hair that match my melting crystal kingdom. My mouth is a raven that haunts Poe, my eyes two slits of labradorite. My caliginous boots beat the pavement, glinting in the insouciant sun …

By the time I escape the plaza, I feel a third of my age—the age I was when I first applied a cheap black lipstick to mimic a goth girl much cooler than me. I was too buoyant (and loud and high-pitched) to ever truly be goth, but my poetic sensibility and low-grade depression felt enough to stand a chance. Though I am no longer young, it's just as exhilarating to experiment with my look. Women over forty are so often exhorted to go "softer" with their palette—as if a cashmere shade of blush or lipstick will blur the lines of a face that has beamed, grimaced, gasped, and laughed; that has screamed, wept, sweat, and sung; that has had the audacity to show up and *live*.

Decades after delivering Avon catalogs and adorning my windowsill with lipstick testers, I no longer scrimp for Sephora brands nor believe that beauty—my own or anyone else's—can save me. I have never, of course, needed to be saved. Whether I'm feeling girly, tough, avant-garde, or all three at the same time, that can manifest in my lip color. A swipe of poppy lightens a heavy day; a pink shimmer counterbalances my natural indignation.

Lipstick may be a small luxury, but its power of reinvention is positively epic. In a world where change is the only constant, a new shade of lipstick openly affirms that "this face, too, is temporary," just as it declares that "this person's story is still being written."

Lipstick's possibilities should be available to anyone curious. May a femme-friendlier future welcome that pleasure.

ACKNOWLEDGMENTS

This book is indebted to the contributions of almost a hundred people, between the ages of ten and seventy-five, who graciously filled out my lipstick questionnaire in 2024, many of whom generously made themselves available for conversation and follow-up questions. These contributors include Leta Harrison, Davon Chance, Tiffany Phillips, Melody Moezzi, Aisha Sultan, Froggi VanRiper, Nora Gruber, JoAnna Novak, Kasey Grady, Barbara G'Sell, Dorris Scott, Sheenu Chacko, Seema Dahlheimer, Temperance Aghamohammadi, Shaela Woody, Kennedy Morganfield, Treasure Shields Redmond, Safa Khatib, Maurice Tracy, Mariama Lockington, Lydia Paar, Louisa Martin, Kaylei Knight, Margaret Keller, Roseann Weiss, René Spencer Saller, Helen Rosner, Bridget Biundo, Meredyth Barr, Smitha Mahesh, Elizabeth Schwartz, Sarah Chiang, Ella English, Livia Xandersmith, Sydney Demchak, Angela Lee, Marcela Fuentes, Rachel Slaughter, Claire Martin, Cynthia Duffy, and Terri Taylor.

I would also like to thank Cynthia Barounis, Tiffany Phillips, Heather Bennett, Temperance Aghamohammadi, and Aisha Sultan for editorial suggestions in the process of creating and revising the first draft; and to librarian extraordinaire Walter Schlect, who guided me through the occasionally byzantine process of seeking out topical popular sources. Thanks to Lucy Jane Santos, Hillary Belzer, and the lovely humans at the Cosmetics History and Makeup Studies Network, who welcomed me despite a lack of historical-scholarship credentials. Thanks to Washington University's Center for Humanities, who granted me access to an office for use on nights and weekends.

Big thank you to Object Lessons editor Christopher Schaberg, who encouraged me to pursue this idea the first day we met in 2023; Kelly Smits for comments and edits on the near-final draft; and Hali Han, at Bloomsbury, for patiently considering my questions on organizing the manuscript. Huge thanks as well to Ari Stern, who not only endured my weekend binge-writing, but lent his prepositional prowess and syntactical sagacity to editing the final draft.

Finally, deep gratitude to all who, at any point, have dared to paint themselves in a way that feels deviant, bold, or magical. This book is for you.

NOTES

Introduction

1 Susan Faludi, *Backlash: The Undeclared War Against American Women* (New York: Three Rivers Press, 1994), 2–3.

2 "Lipstick" today includes lip paint, stain, gloss, oil, ink, and is just as likely to be applied with a wand, brush, or with one's own fingertips. For the purposes of this book, the term "lipstick" applies to all.

3 "Lip cosmetic sales in the United States in 2024, by segment," *Statista*, June 25, 2025, accessed October 18, 2025, https://www.statista.com/statistics/537997/us-lip-cosmetic-sales-by-segment/.

4 "Growth Streak Continues for the US Beauty Industry in 2023," Circana, January 30, 2024, accessed July 24, 2024, https://www.circana.com/intelligence/press-releases/2024/growth-streak-continues-for-the-us-beauty-industry-in-2023-circana-reports/.

5 James Munso, "How Gen Z Is Driving—and Changing—Luxury Beauty," Women's Wear Daily, August 18, 2023, accessed July 24, 2024, https://wwd.com/beauty-industry-news/beauty-features/how-gen-z-is-driving-luxury-beauty-1235763959/.

6 Brooke Sopelsa, "Nearly 30% of Gen Z women identify as LGBTQ, Gallup survey finds," NBC News, March 13, 2024, accessed July 26, 2024, https://www.nbcnews.com/news/us-news/nearly-30-gen-z-women-identify-lgbtq-gallup-survey-finds-rcna143019.

7 Julia Goorin and Rachel Baumgarten, "Insights & Innovation: For Gen Z, Identity is What They Make It," VoxMedia, April 4, 2023, accessed July 26, 2024, https://www.voxmedia.com/2023/4/4/23669479/for-gen-z-identity-is-what-they-make-it.

8 Among books devoted to lipstick itself, Ilise S. Carter's 2021 *The Red Menace: How Lipstick Changed the Face of American History* is the most lively, rigorous, and informative.

9 Meg Cohen Ragas and Karen Kozlowski, *Read My Lips: A Cultural History of Lipstick* (San Francisco: Chronicle Books, 1998), 84.

10 As I wrote in a 2022 essay for *Current Affairs*, this type of "self-care" is hardly the kind of radical affirmation that Black feminist, poet, and civil rights activist Audre Lorde valued in the mid-1980s when she wrote, "Caring for myself is not self-indulgence, it is self-preservation, and that is an act of political warfare."

11 In 2023, the "finger breathing method" received 5.2 million views on TikTok, with users sharing how to breathe and touch their way out of stress and restlessness. When I tried it, I simply became more alert to the crummy condition of my cuticles.

12 Nonbinary and gender-fluid individuals also completed the questionnaires; I indicate their identities where relevant.

13 These vignettes are excerpted from questionnaires.

Chapter 1

1 Dave Kindy, "World's oldest known lipstick found in Iran — a country that banned makeup," *Washington Post*, March 11, 2024, accessed August 9, 2024, https://www.washingtonpost.com/history/2024/03/11/oldest-lipstick-iran/.

2 "Iran's Cosmetics Market on Growth Trajectory," *Financial Tribune*, September 24, 2017, accessed August 9, 2024, https://financialtribune.com/articles/economy/73022/iran-s-cosmetics-market-on-growth-trajectory.

3 Zahra Hankir, *Eyeliner: A History* (New York: Penguin, 2023), 97. While I don't discuss the painting of eyelids in this book, I recommend Hankir's volume for an in-depth discussion of the practice and its significance.

4 Shandiz Moslehi, et al., "Predisposing factors of using cosmetics in Iranian female students: application of prototype willingness model." *Frontiers in Psychology*, 15 (2024): 1381747, accessed August 9, 2024, https://doi.org/10.3389/fpsyg.2024.1381747.

5 "Makeup Survey: Female-Identified Iranian College Students," Survey, YouGov, June 2023, https://d3nkl3psvxxpe9.cloudfront.net/documents/Makeup_poll_results.pdf.

6 Michael D. Lemonick, "Body Art," *Time*, November 29, 1999.

7 Sarah Schaffer, "Reading Our Lips: The History of Lipstick Regulation in Western Seats of Power," *Food & Drug Law Journal* 62, no. 1 (2007): 165.

8 Ibid., 166.

9 Ibid., 166.

10 Ibid., 167.

11 The Poynter Institute corrected the common misperception that the UK actually *did* criminalize lipstick. While there were several attempts to ban it, none were successful. Samantha Putterman, "No, British Parliament Didn't Ban 'Witchcraft' Lipstick in 1770," PolitiFact, October 24, 2019, accessed August 16, 2024, https://www.politifact.com/factchecks/2019/oct/25/facebook-posts/no-british-parliament-didnt-ban-witchcraft-lipstic/.

12 Ilise S. Carter, *Red Menace: How Lipstick Changed the Face of American History* (New York: Prometheus, 2021): 8.

13 Ibid., 8.

14 Ibid., 9.

15 Megan Kessler, "Sparing the 'Angel of the House': Why Victorian Men Used Prostitutes to Avoid Sin," *Historia*, 23 (2014), accessed October 22, 2025, https://www.eiu.edu/historia/Kessler2014.pdf.

16 Jaclyn Reid, "Sex for Sale: Prostitution and Visual Culture, 1850–1910," York University Master's Thesis, 2004, 33.

17 Carter, 18.

18 The Mann Act of 1910, otherwise known as the "White Slave Traffic Act," created federal law against "prostitution or debauchery, or for any other immoral purpose," and essentially drove sex work underground.

19 Carter, 36.

20 Reid, 36.

21 Ibid., 62.

22 Ibid., 63,

23 By now, it was available in "stick" form. The first portable tube was patented in 1915, and did much to encourage its mass consumption; the first swivel-up tube was invented in 1923, around the same time as the rise of the flapper.

24 Reid, 38.

25 Ibid., 39.

26 "Going Hollywood: Movie Fan Magazines," The Henry Ford Museum, February 27, 2014, accessed August 23, 2024, https://www.thehenryford.org/explore/blog/going-hollywood-movie-fan-magazines.

27 "Max Factor: American makeup designer," Encyclopedia Brittanica, updated January 1, 2025. https://www.britannica.com/biography/Max-Factor.

28 Women of color were avid moviegoers in the early 1900s but were generally not represented onscreen. Scholar Richard W. Waterman calls this period the "peak of white supremacy" in terms of media representation. See his "The dark side of the farce: racism in early cinema, 1894–1915," *Politics, Groups, and Identities*, 9, no. 4 (2021): 784–806.

29 It wasn't until the 1964 Civil Rights Act and the 1965 Voting Rights Act that Black, indigenous, Latinx, and other women and men of color were ensured anything close to equal voting rights.

30 "What Beauty Rituals Mean To Me, As An Iranian Woman," *Frenshe,* March 13, 2023. https://frenshe.com/what-beauty-rituals-mean-to-me-as-an-iranian-woman/

31 Farzaneh Milani, "Lipstick Politics in Iran," *New York Times*, August 19, 1999, accessed August 29, 2024, https://www.nytimes.com/1999/08/19/opinion/lipstick-politics-in-iran.html.

32 "Lipstick Revolution: Iranian Women Take to the Streets," ABC News, June 19, 2009, accessed August 29, 2024, https://abcnews.go.com/Politics/International/story?id=7880379.

33 Maryam Foumani, "Two decades of Iranian women's street protests–in pictures," *The Guardian*, October 7, 2022, accessed August 29, 2024, https://www.theguardian.com/global-development/gallery/2022/oct/07/two-decades-of-iranian-womens-street-protests-arash-ashourinia-in-pictures.

Chapter 2

1 Martha J. Bailey and Thomas A. DiPrete, "Five Decades of Remarkable but Slowing Change in U.S. Women's Economic and Social Status and Political Participation," *The Russell Sage Foundation Journal of the Social Sciences* 2, no. 4 (August 2016): 2.

2 Ibid., 3.

3 I recommend Richard Reeves's recent *Of Boys and Men* for a compelling, if disquieting, account of the struggles of men from working class and impoverished backgrounds. Richard Reeves, *Of Boys and Men*, (Washington DC: Brookings Institution Press, 2022).

4 Dennis Hunt, "Behind Poison's Paint," *Los Angeles Times*, April 26, 1987, accessed September 13, 2024, https://www.latimes.com/archives/la-xpm-1987-04-26-ca-1192-story.html.

5 "Working girl" has long been a euphemism for a sex worker.

6 Between the 1960s and 1980s, New York drag competitions known as "balls" gradually evolved into "vogue" battles in Black and Latinx communities. Jennie Livingston's 1990 documentary *Paris Is Burning* captures a glimpse of this vibrant, embattled scene, but is also controversial; Livingston

is white, and none of the voguers depicted in her film were compensated, despite many being working class, poor, or unhoused.

7 Madonna collaborated with choreographers and dancers from the ball scene, like Jose Gutierez and Luis Camacho from the House of Xtravaganza, so she didn't just mimic their moves; she hired them. That said, very little credit was given at the time.

8 Of course, Cher also comes to mind, but wasn't *quite* as popular on Top 40 Radio when I was growing up.

9 The fact that having sex with women instead of men meant lower risk of transmission was hardly passed along.

10 In other justice-related matters, Sephora has not had a perfect record. During the pandemic, massive layoffs shocked thousands of part-time employees. Other lawsuits have been filed for the corporation's failure to consistently pay overtime. "Sephora Employee Calls Out Company's Broken Promises to Part-Timers, Attempts to Buy Workers' Silence," United For Respect, April 20, 2020, https://united4respect.org/press-release/sephora-employee-calls-out-companys-broken-promises-to-part-timers-attempts-to-buy-workers-silence/.

11 I believe the gloss was from an Aussie company called Poppy, that, alas, is no longer sold stateside.

12 Jia Tolentino, "What Tweens Get from Sephora and What They Get from Us," *New Yorker*, August 10, 2024, accessed September 21, 2024, https://www.newyorker.com/culture/the-weekend-essay/what-tweens-get-from-sephora-and-what-they-get-from-us.

13 Becca Rothfeld, *All Things Are Too Small: Essays in Praise of Excess* (New York: Metropolitan, 2024), 37.

14 Ibid., 38.

15 "You Look Good," Glossier, YouTube, October 11, 2022, https://www.youtube.com/watch?v=m-5VU1pnTb0.

16 Diana Heald, "Gaslight, Gatekeep, Glossier: On Marisa Meltzer's *Glossy*, *Los Angeles Review of Books*, June 8, 2024, accessed September 22, 2024, https://lareviewofbooks.org/article/gaslight-gatekeep-glossier-on-marisa-meltzers-glossy/.

17 Devon Abelman, "Best Lip Paints," *Allure*, March 17, 2017, accessed September 22, 2024, https://www.allure.com/gallery/best-lip-paints.

18 "About Us," Haus Labs, January 9, 2025, https://www.hauslabs.com/pages/about.

19 Ciara Cremin, *Man-Made Woman: The Dialectics of Cross-Dressing*. London: Pluto Press, 73–4.

20 Ibid., 71–2.

Sidebar #1: The Pesky Endurance of Public High School Lipstick Bans

1 Ilise S. Carter, *The Red Menace: How Lipstick Changed the Face of American History*, (New York: Prometheus, 2021), 43.

2 Ibid., 44.

3 Ibid., 45.

4 "Loe. vs. Texas," ACLU, October 18, 2024, https://www.aclu.org/cases/loe-v-texas.

5 Galen Sherwin, Linda Morris, and Eleanor Wachtel, "4 Things Public Schools Can and Can't Do When It Comes to Dress Codes," ACLU, September 21, 2022, accessed October 5, 2024, https://www.aclu.org/news/womens-rights/4-things-public-schools-can-and-cant-do-dress-codes.

Chapter 3

1 Rebecca Onion, "A Modern Feminist Classic Changed My Life. Was It Actually Garbage?" *Slate*, March 30, 2021. "Wolf the star feminist and Wolf the science denouncer share an animating principle: the tendency to feel strongly about something, then decide that the intensity of those feelings means that there must be somebody responsible."

2 Journalist Yvonne Abraham wielded the term "lipstick feminism" as an epithet in a piece for the *Boston Phoenix*. Jennifer Baumgardner and Amy Richards, *Manifesta: Young Women, Feminism, and the Future* (New York: Farrar, Straus and Giroux, 2000), 255.

3 Lauren Gurrieri and Jenna Drenten, "The feminist politics of choice: Lipstick as a Marketplace Icon," *Consumption Markets & Culture* 24, no. 3, 2021: 225. https://doi.org/10.1080/10253866.2019.1670649.

4 Linda M. Scott, *Fresh Lipstick: Redressing Fashion and Feminism*, (New York: Palgrave-MacMillan, 2005), 2–3.

5 Ibid., 2.

6 Ibid., 9.

7 Carter, 17. E. Lynn Linton (1822–98) was Britain's first salaried woman journalist and a Victorian public intellectual. Her essay "The Girl of the Period," from the *Saturday Review*,

was republished in American newspapers and magazines, often without granting her authorial credit. When the essays were republished by the *Saturday Review* in 1883, Linton's preface acknowledged the controversy over her essay decades earlier, writing, "The Girl of the Period" was especially obnoxious to many to whom women were the Sacred Sex above criticism and beyond rebuke; and I had to pay pretty smartly in private life, by those who knew, for what they termed a libel and an untruth. With these passionate repudiators on the one hand, on the other were some who, trading on the enforced anonymity of the paper, took spurious credit to themselves for the authorship." https://www.gutenberg.org/files/41735/41735-h/41735-h.htm#Page_109.

8 Ibid., 7 (italics mine).

9 Scott, 1.

10 Ibid., 2.

11 Sophie Lewis, "Some Like It Hot: Notes from the Marilyn Appreciation Society," *Harper's*, November 2022, accessed October 12, 2024, https://harpers.org/archive/2022/11/some-like-it-hot-notes-from-the-marilyn-appreciation-society/.

12 "Case study: Always #LikeAGirl," Campaign, October 12, 2015, https://www.campaignlive.co.uk/article/case-study-always-likeagirl/1366870.

13 AD Wonk, "This is an Ad for Men," YouTube, March 21, 2021, 02:21, https://www.youtube.com/watch?v=jdyym9hnbPU.

14 Scott, 241.

15 Andi Ziesler, *We Were Feminists Once: From Riot Grrrl to CoverGirl, the Buying and Selling of a Political Movement* (New York: Public Affairs, 2016), xv.

16 John Berger, *Ways of Looking*, (New York: Penguin, 1977), 47.

17 Judith Butler, *Gender Trouble: Feminism and the Subversion of Identity* (New York: Routledge, 1990).

18 Ibid., 25.

19 Becca Rothfeld, *All Things Are Too Small: Essays in Praise of Excess*, (New York: MacMillan, 2024), 216–17.

20 Ibid., 217.

21 Jack Halberstam, *Gaga Feminism: Sex, Gender, and the End of Normal*, (New York: Beacon Press, 2013), 25.

22 Ibid., 12.

23 Ibid., 12.

24 Ibid., 11.

25 Ibid., 13.

26 Ibid., 13.

27 Ibid., 15.

28 Beverly D'Silva, "How Iris Apfel became an icon in her 90s," BBC, March 2, 2024, accessed October 26, 2024, https://www.bbc.com/culture/article/20240302-how-iris-apfel-became-an-icon-in-her-90s.

29 Halberstam, 10.

30 During her audition for the former film, director Bradley Cooper commanded that Gaga "take it off"—the "it" meaning her face full of makeup—as he wanted to see her "completely open" and with "no artifice." Evidently, he took it upon himself to pull out a makeup wipe and remove it himself (an act that, frankly, resembles a form of assault).

Sidebar #2: The Myth of the Red-Lipped Suffragette

1 Jessica Pallingston, *Lipstick: A Celebration of the World's Favorite Cosmetic* (New York: St. Martin's Press, 1999), 15.

2 For a fairly quick, yet comprehensive view of photographs chronicling suffrage rallies, the following link is helpful: https://www.theatlantic.com/photo/2019/06/the-battle-for-womens-suffrage-in-photos/591103/.

3 Lucy Jane Santos, "History of Lipstick: Elizabeth Arden Red," *Past to Present with Lucy Jane Santos*, August 23, 2023, accessed October 12, 2024, https://lucyjanesantos.com/2024/08/23/elizabeth-arden-and-the-red-lipstick-that-wasnt/.

4 Linda M. Scott, *Fresh Lipstick: Redressing Fashion and Feminism* (Palgrave: 2005), 137.

5 Santos.

6 "U.N. Women," unwomen.org, accessed October 22, 2025, https://www.unwomen.org/en.

Chapter 4

1 Michelle Lavergne, "'Black Girls Don't Wear Red Lipstick' Exhibit Challenges Beauty Standards," *Reporting Texas*, February 16, 2024, accessed October 19, 2024, https://www.reportingtexas.com/black-girls-dont-wear-red-lipstick-exhibit-challenges-beauty-standards/.

2 Johanna Ferreria, "Why I'm Reclaiming Red Lipstick as a Latina," Thirteen Lune, accessed October 30, 2024. https://

thirteenlune.com/blogs/shop-talk/why-i-m-reclaiming-red-lipstick-as-a-latina.

3 Chloe Benson, "The (Dis)Invention of Black Women: A Rhetorical Analysis of Intersectional Oppression within Cosmetics Practices," *Veritas: Villanova Research Journal* 3 no. 1, January 14, 2022.

4 Medina Azaldin, "History of the Hero: MAC Ruby Woo Lipstick," *Harper's Bazaar*, November 22, 2022, https://www.harpersbazaar.com/uk/beauty/make-up-nails/a41886695/mac-ruby-woo-lipstick/.

5 Andrea Arterbery, "The Invisible Woman: A Study of Black Women In Magazine Beauty Advertisement." Master of the Arts, Thesis, University of North Texas, May 2019, 3, https://mocada.org/dissertation-the-invisible-woman/

6 Alicia Vitarelli, "Temple grad Camille Bell's inclusive Pound Cake lipstick line sells out overnight," 6ABC Philadelphia, October 29, 2021, accessed October 22, 2025, https://6abc.com/post/pound-cake-lipstick-inclusive-temple-university-graduate/11181006/.

7 Brandon Patterson, "Detroit-launched Lip Bar goes from 'Shark Tank' rejection to Target," *Detroit Free Press*, February 23, 2018. https://www.freep.com/story/money/business/2018/02/23/lip-bar-shark-tank-target/358520002/

8 "Kevin: Lip Bar Is Clown Makeup," *Shark Tank*, Season 6, Week 17, 2015, accessed October 12, 2024, https://abc.com/video/09b810db-4142-4e8c-9e18-d637a0c86c8a

9 Brandon Patterson, "Detroit-launched Lip Bar goes from 'Shark Tank' rejection to Target," *Detroit Free Press*, February 23, 2018, accessed October 26, 2024, https://www.freep.com/story/money/business/2018/02/23/lip-bar-shark-tank-target/358520002/.

10 Kristin Denise Row, "'Unmanageable': Exploring Black Girlhood, Storytelling, and Ideas of Beauty," *Open Cultural Studies*, 6, no. 1 (October 2022): 243–59.

11 Heather Radke's *Butts: A Backstory* does an excellent job unpacking the racialized nature of the derriere across Western history and aesthetics. Heather Radke, *Butts: A Backstory*, (New York: Simon & Schuster, 2022).

12 Qtd. Carter, *The Red Menace*, 65.

13 Maxine Leeds Craig, "Black Women and Beauty Culture in 20th-Century America." *Oxford Research Encyclopedia of American History*, November 20, 2017, accessed September 7, 2025, https://oxfordre.com/americanhistory/view/10.1093/acrefore/9780199329175.001.0001/acrefore-9780199329175-e-433.

14 Although Madam C. J. Walker refused to sell skin bleaching products, following her death in 1919, and under pressure to compete in the drugstore market, the company introduced a bleaching cream, which quickly became their bestselling product.

15 Melissa L. Baird, "Making Black More Beautiful: Black Women and the Cosmetics Industry in the Post-Civil Rights Era," *Gender & History* 33, no. 2 (July 2021), 559.

16 Camille Wise, "'Gurl, Yo Foundation Don't Match': 40 Years of African American Makeup in *Ebony* Magazine," University Honors Thesis, California State University, Long Beach, Spring 2020, http://hdl.handle.net/20.500.12680/8910k096r.

17 Baird, 561.

18 Ibid., 571.

19 Johanna Ferreria, "Why I'm Reclaiming Red Lipstick as a Latina," *Thirteen Lune*, accessed November 9, 2024, https://thirteenlune.com/blogs/shop-talk/why-i-m-reclaiming-red-lipstick-as-a-latina.

20 Madison Feller, "Alexandria Ocasio-Cortez Knows She Can't Save America All by Herself," *Elle*, July 16, 2018, https://www.elle.com/culture/career-politics/a22118408/alexandria-ocasio-cortez-interview/.

21 Mónica G. Moreno Figueroa, "Picking your Battles: Beauty, Complacency, and the Other Life of Racism," in *The Routledge Companion to Beauty Politics*, ed. M.L. Craig (London: Routledge, 2021), 53.

22 Ayesha Le Breton, "The South Asian History of Red," *The Juggernaut*, December 19, 2023, accessed November 9, 2024, https://www.thejuggernaut.com/red-history-importance-in-south-asia.

23 Rajika Puri, "Bharatanatyam Performed: A Typical Recital," *Visual Anthropology* 17, no. 1 (January 2004): 173.

24 Ibid., 176.

25 Jia Tolentino, "The Age of Instagram Face," *The New Yorker*, December 12, 2019, accessed November 9, 2024, https://www.newyorker.com/culture/decade-in-review/the-age-of-instagram-face.

26 "Lip Augmentation Market Size, Share & Trends Analysis Report by Type (Temporary, Permanent), by Product (Hyaluronic Acid Fillers, Lip Collagen), by Region, and Segment Forecasts, 2023–2030," Grand View Research., accessed November 16, 2024, https://www.grandviewresearch.com/industry-analysis/lip-augmentation-market.

27 Zing Tsjeng, "What We Learned from the UK's Biggest Poll About Lip Fillers," *Vice*, October 2, 2019, accessed November 16, 2024, https://www.vice.com/en/article/lip-fillers-uk-opinion-poll/.

28 "United States: Lip Augmentation Attitudes in 2017, by Ethnicity." *Statista*, June 22, 2017, accessed November

17, 2024, https://www.statista.com/statistics/724397/lip-augmentation-attitudes-of-americans-by-ethnicity/.

29 Nadine Palmer, "Did Kim Kardashian steal from Black culture to build her body, brands and profit? New study investigated," Brunel University, May 22 2024, accessed November 24, 2024, https://www.brunel.ac.uk/news-and-events/news/articles/Did-Kim-Kardashian-steal-from-Black-culture-to-build-her-body-brands-and-profit-New-study-investigated.

30 Adrienne Santos-Longhurst, "How Much Do Lip Fillers Cost? Average Cost by Location and Brand," March 29, 2024, accessed November 24, 2024, https://www.carecredit.com/well-u/health-wellness/lip-fillers-cost.

31 L. Smith, "Leta Harrison: A Historical Love Letter to Black Womens' Boldness," *Austin Woman*, March 1, 2024, accessed October 22, 2025, https://atxwoman.com/2024/03/01/see-her-work-leta-harrison/.

Sidebar #3: Four Decades of Lipstick Lyrics and Music Videos

1 Suzi Quatro, "Lipstick," YouTube, February 15, 2015, 4:09, https://www.youtube.com/watch?v=DAPfFfsrzm0.

2 Tori Amos, "Cornflake Girl," YouTube, January 10, 2014, 3:55, https://www.youtube.com/watch?v=w_HA5Czhtx4.

3 Eve's Plum, "Lipstuck Lyrics," Genius, https://genius.com/Eves-plum-lipstuck-lyrics.

4 Ashley Spencer, "What Happened to Vitamin C?" *Vice*, September 17, 2019, accessed November 18, 2024, https://www.vice.com/en/article/what-happened-to-vitamin-c-singer-of-graduation-and-smile-2019/.

5 Janelle Monae, "Lipstick Lover," YouTube, May 11, 2023, 3:26, https://www.youtube.com/watch?v=Y7S6wLP_vsY.

6 "Chappell Roan: Tiny Desk Concert," YouTube, March 21, 2024, 23:01, https://www.youtube.com/watch?v=w4WiXKGCJhg.

7 James Factora, "Here's How to Recreate Chappell Roan's Camp-Meets-Couture Tiny Desk Look," *Them*, March 26, 2024, accessed November 18, 2024, https://www.them.us/story/how-to-recreate-chappell-roans-npr-tiny-desk-makeup-look.

Chapter 5

1 Chappell Roan, "yes i took a full chomp out of the bundle of lipstick…" Instagram, August 19, 2024, https://www.instagram.com/chappellroan/p/C-2j5UqJ2XD/?hl=en&img_index=1.

2 I do not mean to suggest that *all* of "BimboTok" is feminist, or that "Bimbo feminism" is necessarily progressive, but agree with queer feminist Sophie Lewis who deems that "theirs is an ethos that posits machismo and femmephobia as two sides of the same coin." Sophie Lewis, "Some Like It Hot," *Harper's*, November 22, 2024.

3 Alex Berg, "Why My Lipstick is My Queer Armor," *Them*, February 5, 2018, accessed January 4, 2025, https://www.them.us/story/why-lipstick-is-my-queer-armor.

4 Nicole Dall'Asen, "Ilona Maher's $10 Lipstick Doesn't Budge, Even In Head-On Rugby Collisions," *Allure*, July 31, 2024, accessed January 4, 2025, https://www.allure.com/story/ilona-maher-2024-olympics-beauty-routine.

5 YouGov Survey, June 23–27, 2023. https://d3nkl3psvxxpe9.cloudfront.net/documents/Makeup_poll_results.pdf

6 This survey focuses on white women from the South and West regions of the US, with a fairly even split politically between parties. Sexual identity and orientation were not surveyed.

7 Alexandra Sifferlin, "Science Shows Men Like Women with Less Makeup," *Time*, April 29, 2014, accessed January 5, 2025, https://time.com/79584/science-women-less-makeup/.

8 Alex L. Jones, Robin S. S. Kramer, and Robert Ward. "Miscalibrations in Judgements of Attractiveness with Cosmetics," *Quarterly Journal of Experimental Psychology* 67, no. 10, 2014, 2060–68.

9 Martha Mills, "Men like women to wear less makeup? No, they don't," *The Guardian*, March 23, 2016, January 6, 2025, https://www.theguardian.com/science/brain-flapping/2016/mar/23/men-women-less-makeup-bad-research.

10 In a fascinating 2021 psychology study from Goldsmiths, University of London, it was discovered that straight men who unwittingly express attraction toward trans women compensate by adhering to stronger anti-gay sentiments. West, Keon, and Martha Lucia Borras-Guevara. "When Cisgender, Heterosexual Men Feel Attracted to Transgender Women: Sexuality-Norm Violations Lead to Compensatory Anti-Gay Prejudice," *Journal of Homosexuality* 69, no. 13 (2022): 2267–85.

11 Jenn Hunter, "Jeffree Star's Net Worth: How Much Money Does the Shocking YouTube Beauty Influencer and Brand Owner Have?" *Capitalism*, July 7, 2023, https://www.capitalism.com/jeffree-stars-net-worth/.

12. Daphné B., *Made-Up: A True Story of Beauty Culture Under Late Capitalism,* Toronto: Coach House Books, 2020, 32.

13. Ibid., 42.

14. Ibid., 12.

INDEX